W9-AAH-604

# HOW YOUR HEART WORKS

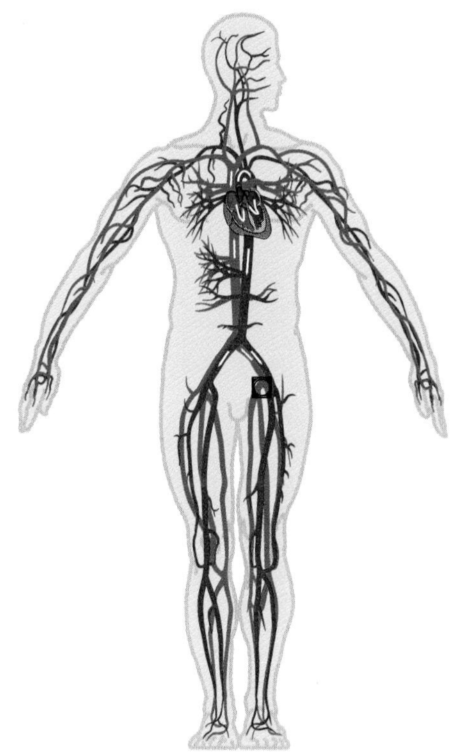

*HOW YOUR HEART WORKS* DESCRIBES THE HUMAN CARDIOVASCULAR SYSTEM IN GENERAL AND DISCUSSES MANY COMMON CONDITIONS AND DISORDERS. IT TRIES TO MAKE YOU A SMARTER CONSUMER OF HEALTH SERVICES AND PRODUCTS, BUT IT DOES NOT OFFER MEDICAL ADVICE AND IS NOT A SUBSTITUTE FOR MEDICAL CARE OR SUPERVISION. CONSULT A PHYSICIAN ABOUT ALL YOUR SPECIFIC HEALTH CONCERNS.

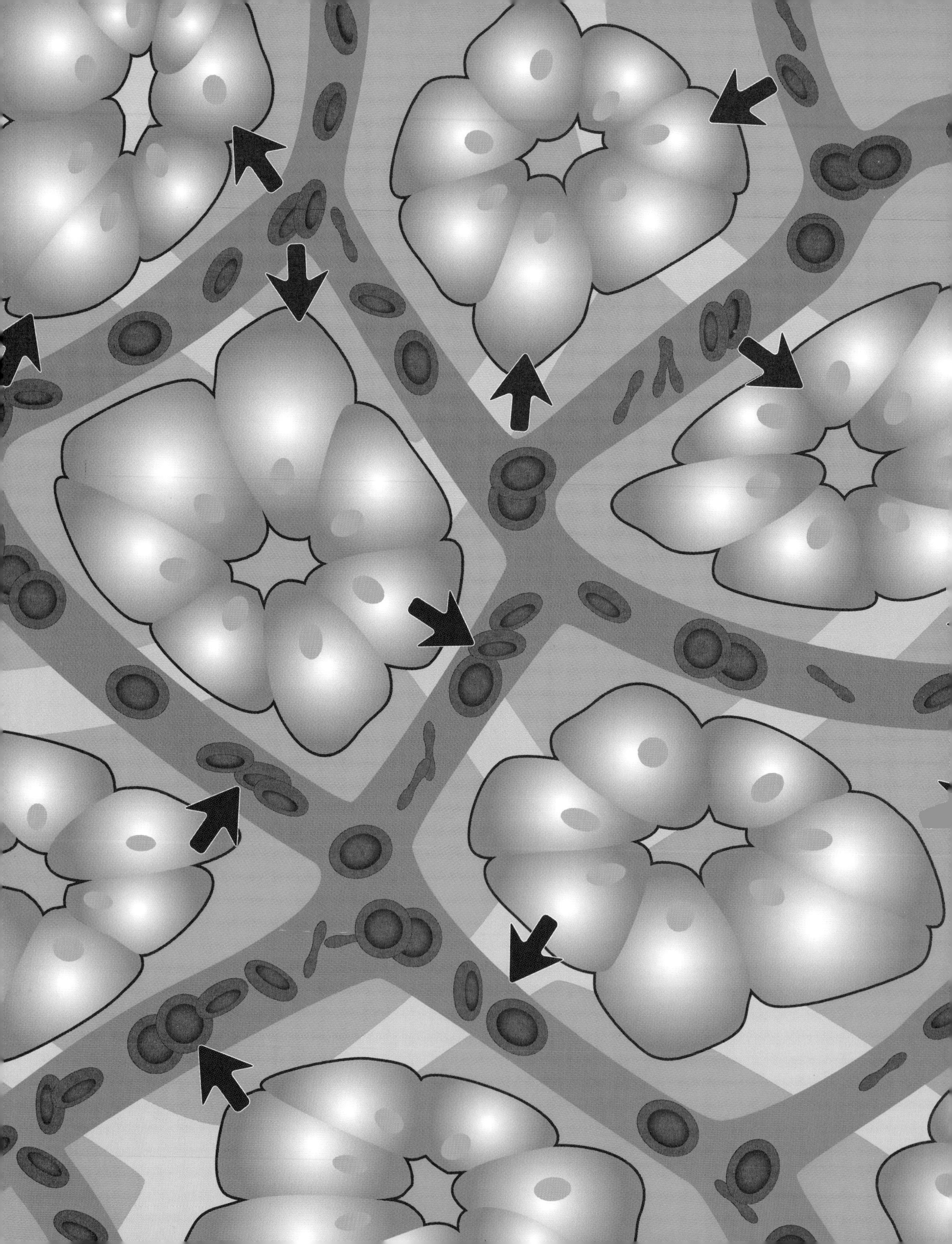

# HOW YOUR HEART WORKS

RALPH MYERSON, M.D.

Illustrated by

DOUGLAS BECKNER

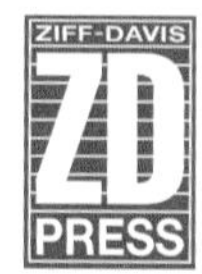


Ziff-Davis Press

Emeryville, California

| | |
|---|---|
| Editor | Ann Donaldson |
| Technical Reviewers | Claudia Prose, M.D., and Howard Savage, M.D. |
| Project Coordinator | Barbara Dahl |
| Proofreader | Carol Burbo |
| Cover Illustration | Regan Honda and Douglas Beckner |
| Cover Design | Regan Honda |
| Book Design | Carrie English |
| Technical Illustration | Douglas Beckner |
| Word Processing | Howard Blechman |
| Page Layout | Tony Jonick |
| Indexer | Valerie Robbins |

Ziff-Davis Press books are produced on a Macintosh computer system with the following applications: FrameMaker®, Microsoft® Word, QuarkXPress®, Adobe Illustrator®, Adobe Photoshop®, Adobe Streamline™, MacLink®*Plus*, Aldus® FreeHand™, Collage Plus™.

If you have comments or questions or would like to receive a free catalog, call or write:
Ziff-Davis Press
5903 Christie Avenue
Emeryville, CA 94608
1-800-688-0448


PART OF A CONTINUING SERIES



ISBN 1-56276-238-9

Manufactured in the United States of America
♻ This book is printed on paper that contains 50% total recycled fiber of which 20% is de-inked postconsumer fiber.
10 9 8 7 6 5 4 3 2 1

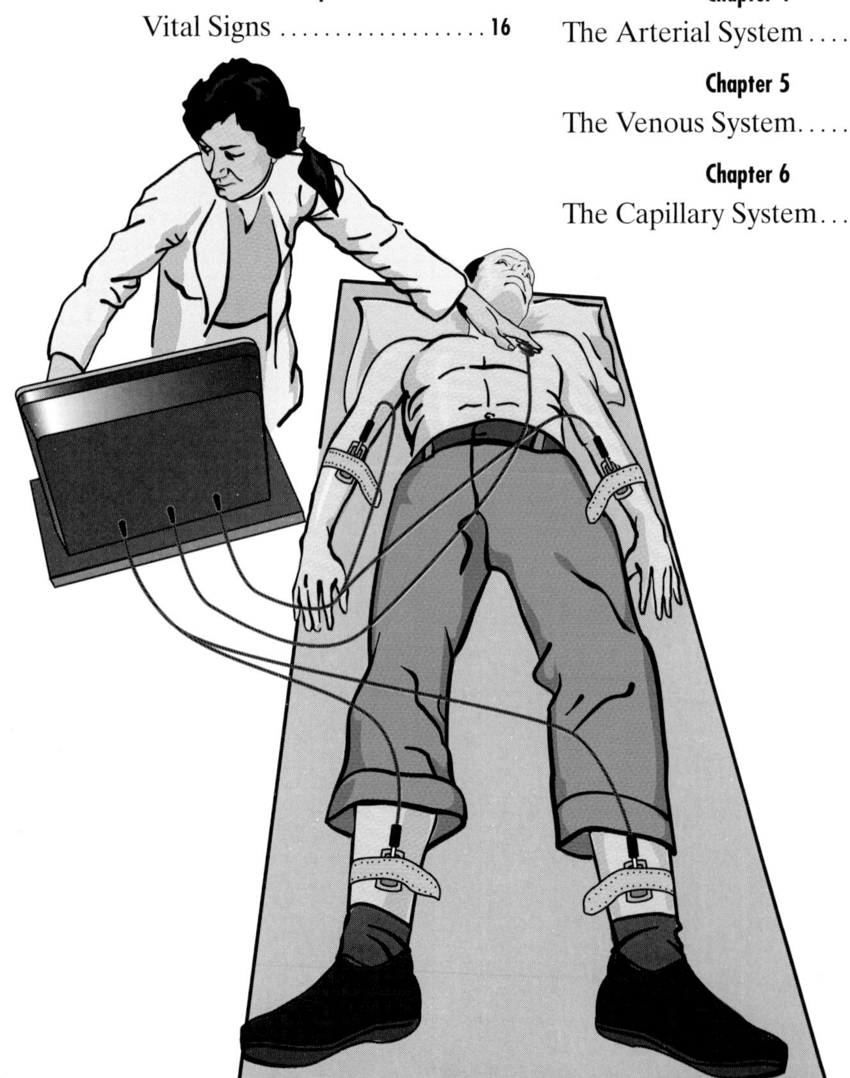

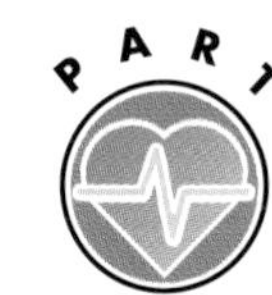

## The Abnormal Heart
70



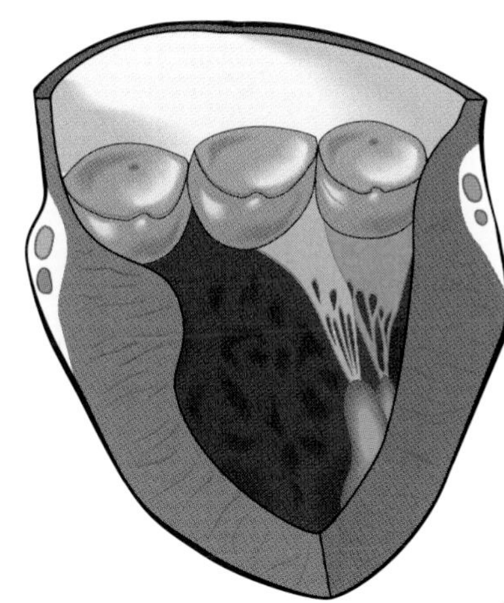

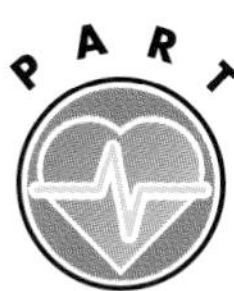

## The Abnormal Vascular System
114



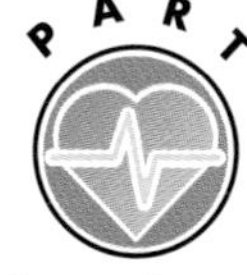

## Cardiopulmonary Resuscitation (CPR)
146



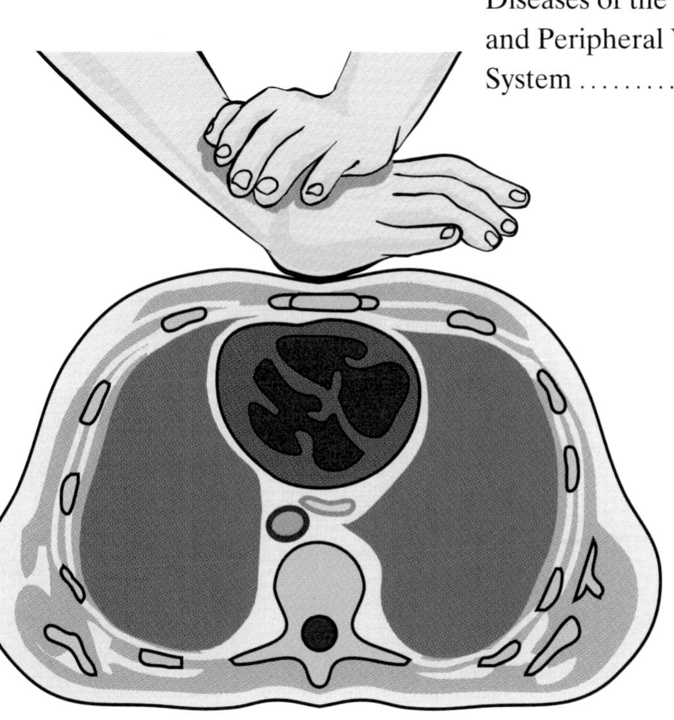

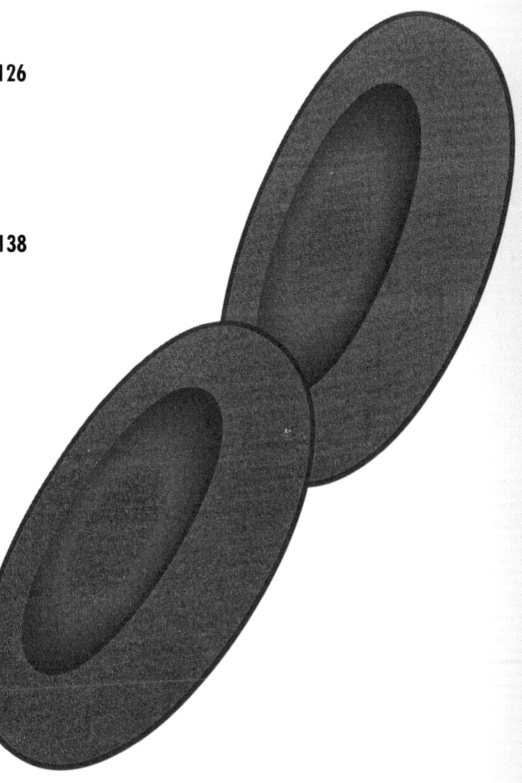

This book would not have been possible without the skillful artistic talents of Doulgas Beckner. I am also grateful to Dr. Claudia Prose for the excellent technical advice she supplied, which helped tremendously in filling the gaps in my knowledge. Many at Ziff-Davis Press provided me with sorely needed writing assistance. Last, but not least, I appreciate the critique provided by my non-medical text reviewers—my wife, Loretta, and my grandchildren, Samuel and Exie Huntington.

There are noticeable gaps in the knowledge of many individuals on the anatomy and functions of the organs of the human body. In fact, there appears to be more awareness of the structure of the atom or the surface of the moon than there is concerning the contraction of the heart and the circulation of the blood. Although educators increaingly are providing students with important knowledge of our body and how it works, a need for such information still exists in a large segment of our population. *How Your Heart Works* is a book that anyone can use to learn more about the inner workings of the heart and blood vessels—the cardiovascular system. Perhaps you or someone you know has been diagnosed with a heart problem and you'd like to know more about how the cardiovascular system works. Or maybe you, like thousands of others, have always been interested in how the human body works but have not been able to find a resource written in plain English that provides the essential information you want

*How Your Heart Works* attempts to fill the void in knowledge that is present concerning the cardiovascular system. In it you'll find a unique combination of words and illustrations that not only guide you through the anatomy and function of the normal heart and vascular system (the veins, arteries, and capillaries), but also show you what happens when the cardiovascular system does not work properly. Along the way you see how patient and physician can work together to keep the heart healthy and to reach a diagnosis and treatment plan if needed. You'll see how technological tools such as the electrocardiogram, CAT scan, and MRI work. The last chapter illustrates the life-saving technique of cardiopulmonary resuscitation (CPR), giving you the knowledge to assist in a cardiovascular emergency.

*How Your Heart Works* is dedicated to educating its readers. It is not intended to be a book for self-diagnosis and treatment and does not take the place of the physician. Readers should continue to consult their physicians for their medical needs.

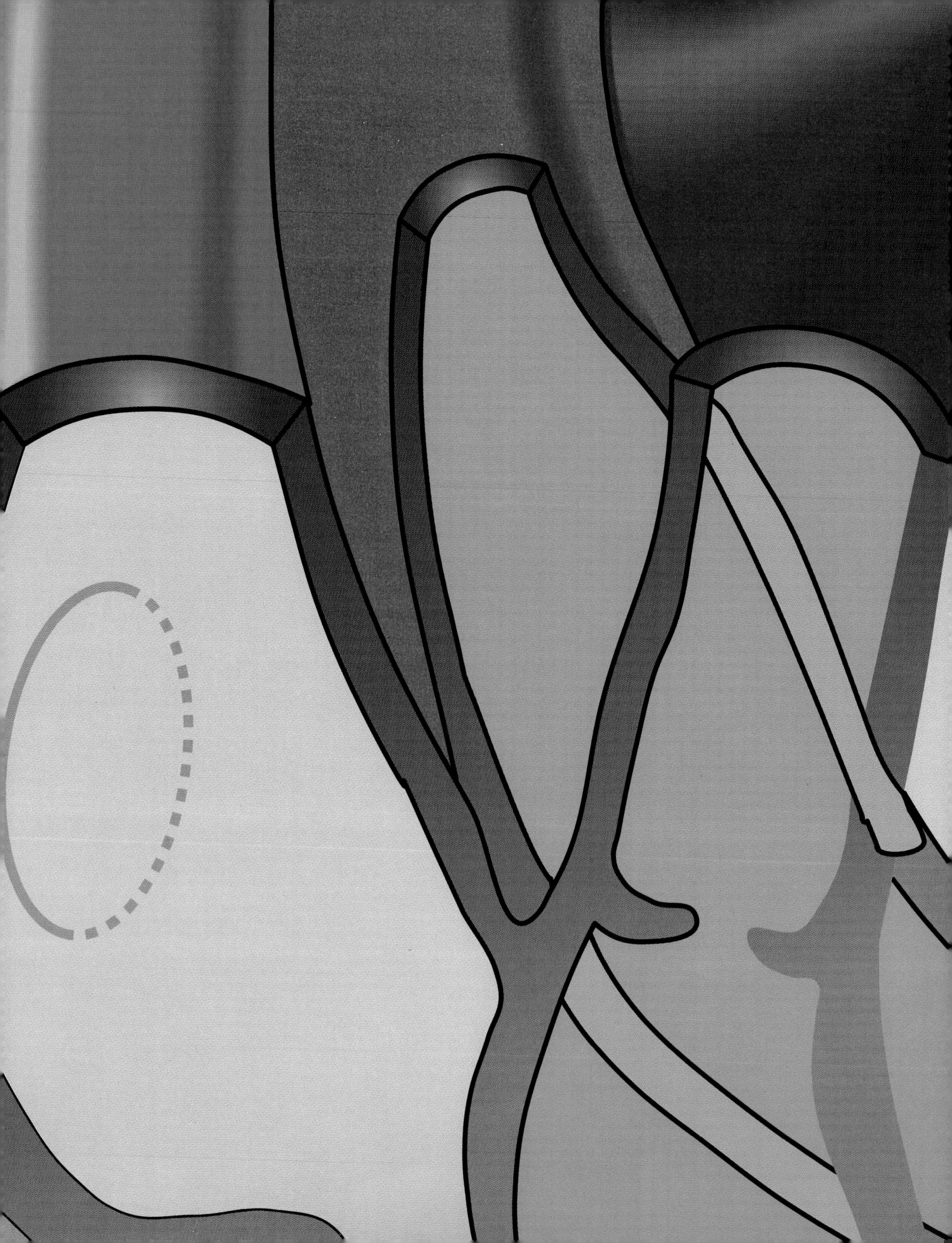

PART 1

# THE NORMAL HEART: A FANTASTIC PUMP

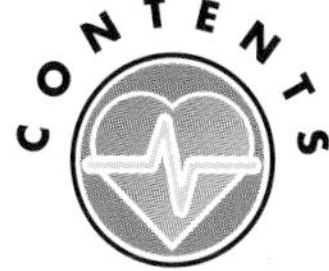

THE MORE WE know about how our hearts work, the better we can appreciate what an amazing organ it is.

Although our ancestors were unaware of the real function of the heart, they did know that it was vital and central to their existence. It was not until the early seventeenth century that we were given the first glimpse into the intricate workings of the heart. At that time, William Harvey, the court physician of King Charles I of England, conducted human and animal experiments that defined the pumping role of the heart, the role of the blood vessels, and the flow from the heart through the blood vessels and back to the heart. In 1628, he published his treatise, *On the Movement of the Heart and Blood,* and the concepts of the heart and the circulatory system were changed forever.

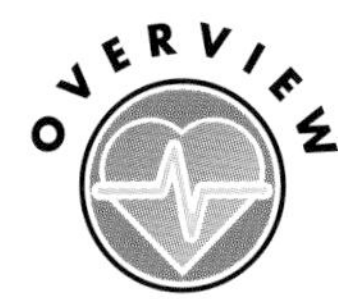


Paradoxically, even after Harvey's monumental work, the medieval notion that the heart was the "noblest of the body organs" and the seat and origin of many emotions and personality traits persisted. Even to this day, we have assigned a number of fanciful attributes to the heart. Thus, the heart is associated with bravery (lionhearted), cruelty (cold-blooded), generosity (big-hearted), sadness (brokenhearted), etc. Of course, its association with love and romance is especially noteworthy. The heart is not only the target for Cupid's arrows, but suffers many, sometimes frightening, indignities in song and poem. We hear of hearts that stand still, break, or bleed. Fortunately, events such as this are not supported by fact.

The heart has been the subject of a vast amount of basic and clinical research, resulting in the accumulation of much important information and the development of crucial technical advances. These advances have enabled us to obtain a thorough understanding of the heart and its functions; diagnosis and treatment of heart ailments are now much better. Over the last few decades, there has been a striking decrease of deaths due to heart disease—the leading cause of death in the United States and the Western world.

Stated in the simplest of terms, the heart is merely a pump, albeit a remarkable one and unparalleled in nature or by human hands. As with most pumps, the function of the heart is to transport a liquid from one place to another. Of course, in the case of the heart, the liquid is blood, the life-sustaining fluid essential for almost every cell, tissue, and organ in the body. Blood carries nutrients and other essential substances, but its most important component is oxygen. Oxygen is vital; if it is absent for four or more minutes, death may result.

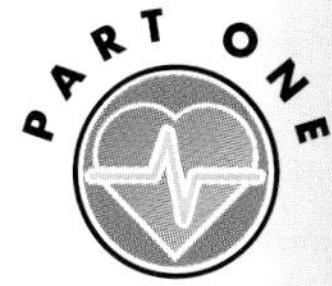


In Part 1 of this book, we get to the heart of the matter and discuss some of the fundamental characterisitics of the organ—its anatomy, its physiology, and how its action is reflected in physical vital signs such as blood pressure, pulse, and cardiac output.

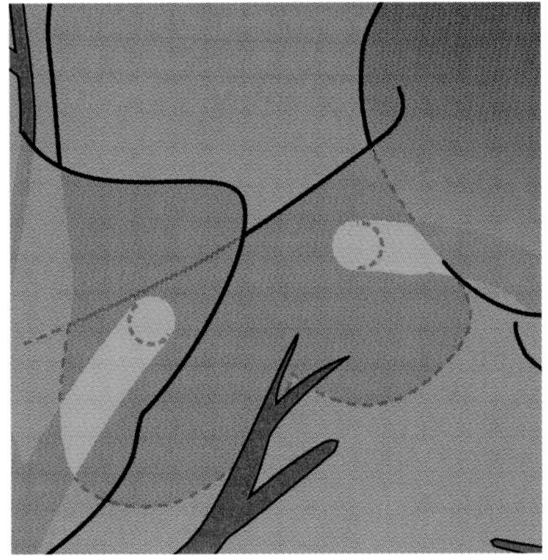

# The Anatomy of the Heart

THE SHAPE OF the human heart bears little resemblance to the one representing St. Valentine's Day. Instead, its shape is more conical with the narrow end pointing downward, to the left and slightly forward. Its location in the chest cavity is just to the left of the midline, behind the sternum and the second to sixth left ribs.

Despite its heavy work load, the human heart is not a large organ; it is about the size of a clenched fist and weighs 10 to 12 ounces. It is surrounded by a membranous sac, the *pericardial sac*, (*peri* means around; *cardia* is from the Greek word for heart, *kardia*). This sac contains a small amount of watery fluid that bathes the heart and protects it from contact with adjacent organs during its contractions.

The wall of the heart consists of three layers of tissue: the *pericardium*, a thin, transparent layer covering the outside of the heart; a similar thin layer, the *endocardium* (*endo* means inner), lining the heart cavity; and a thick layer of cardiac muscle, the *myocardium* (*myo* means muscle), that separates the two linings. The myocardium is a specialized type of muscle that is unique to the heart and responsible for its contractions.

The heart has two thin-walled receiving chambers: the left and right *atria,* and two thick-walled pumping chambers, the *ventricles*. Actually, the heart consists of two parallel pumps that work simultaneously—the right-side pump receives blood from the veins and pumps it to the lungs where it is resupplied with oxygen, and the left-side pump receives the freshly reoxygenated blood from the lungs and sends it through the arteries to the rest of the body. The heart also has four valves. There are two valves between the atria and ventricles to prevent backflow or regurgitation of blood resulting from the high pressure of the ventricular pump action, and two valves to prevent backflow into the ventricles after they have finished their pumping action.

Let's trace the one-way flow of blood through the heart. Blood enters the right atrium from the veins and passes through the *tricuspid* valve into the right ventricle. The right ventricle contracts, expelling blood through the *pulmonic valve* and sending it to the lungs for a fresh supply of oxygen. As the right ventricle contracts, the tricuspid valve snaps shut, preventing regurgitation of blood into the right atrium. As the right ventricle relaxes, the pulmonic valve closes, preventing regurgitation of blood back into the ventricle. The fresh blood from the lungs returns to the heart into the left atrium that passes it into the powerful left ventricle through the *mitral* or *bicuspid valve.* The left ventricle now contracts, sending blood out of the heart through the *aortic valve* into the largest artery in the body, the *aorta.* As the left ventricle contracts, the mitral valve closes, preventing regurgitation of blood from the left ventricle into the left atrium. As the left ventricle relaxes, the aortic valve closes, preventing regurgitation from the aorta back into the left ventricle. This is the way that both sides of the heart, the two atria and the two ventricles, work simultaneously.

Although the heart can operate on its own, it is supplied with two sets of nerves to augment the work. The *sympathetic* nerves stimulate the heart and the *parasympathetic* nerves (mainly the *vagus* nerve) act to calm the heart down. These nervous systems carry signals from the brain and elsewhere in the body that help the heart respond and adjust to internal and external factors. They act chiefly by adjusting the rate at which the heart beats. They are also useful as the mechanism by which many drugs exert their therapeutic effects on the heart by stimulating or blocking the sympathetic or parasympathetic nerves.

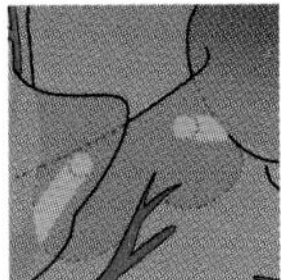

The heart also has its own important blood supply, the *coronary circulation.* The two main coronary arteries, left and right, branch from the aorta just as it leaves the heart. They, in turn, give rise to numerous branches, guaranteeing the heart a rich supply of blood and oxygen. A decrease in the oxygen supply to the heart usually occurs as a result of narrowing or complete obstruction of one or more coronary arteries. When a portion of the myocardium is deprived of oxygen, that portion of the heart muscle may die, a condition known as a *myocardial infarction.* (This will be discussed further later in the book.)

# Anatomy of the Heart

## View of the Heart from Front

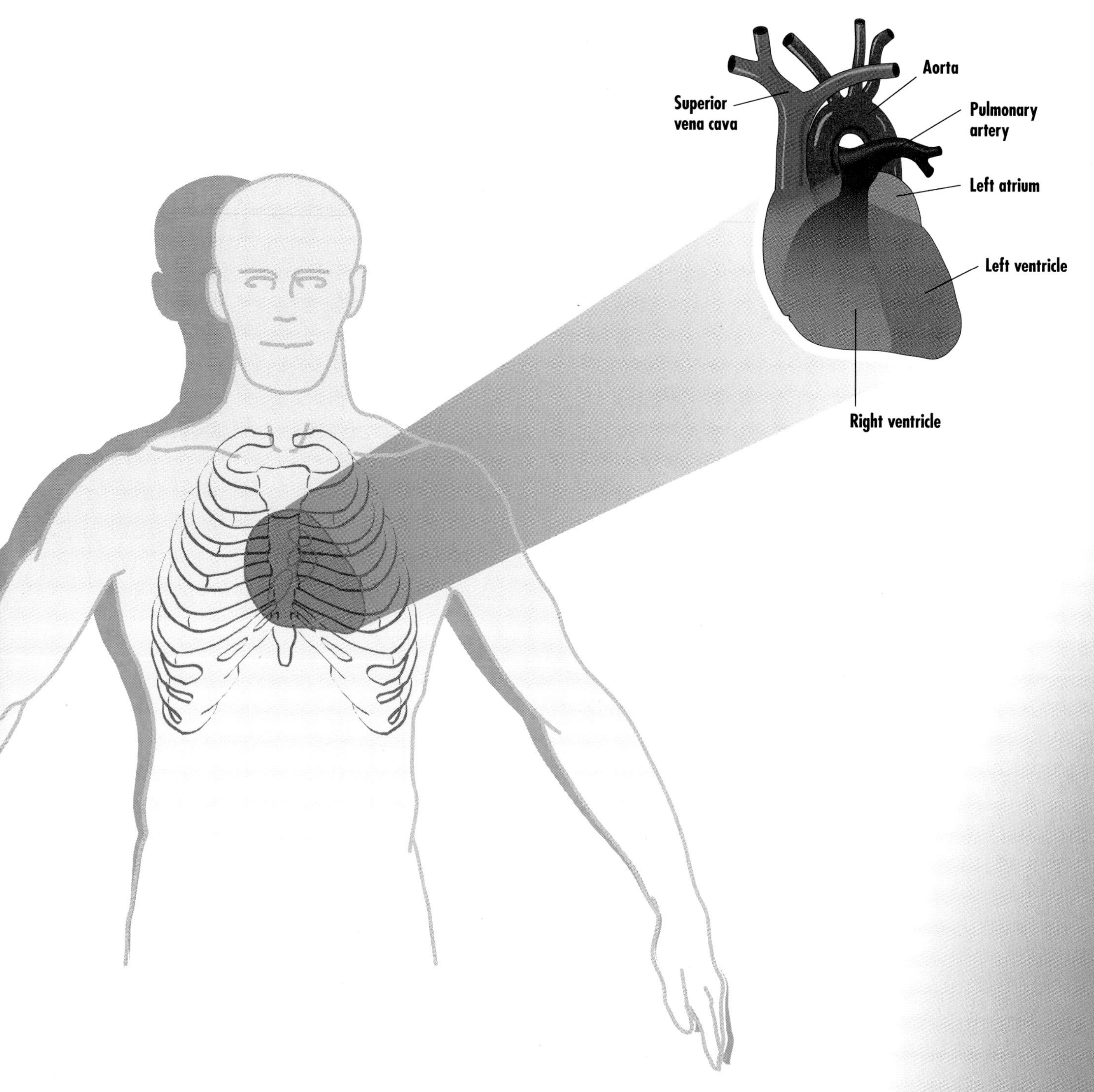

## Chambers and Valves of the Heart

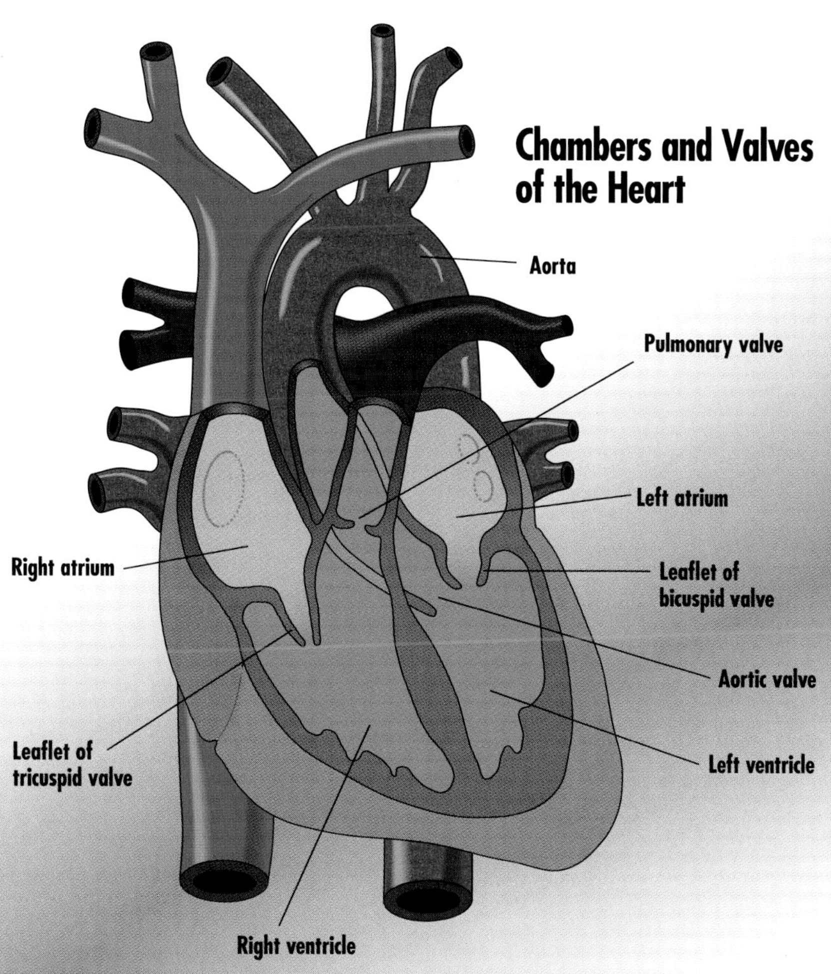


## Coronary Circulation

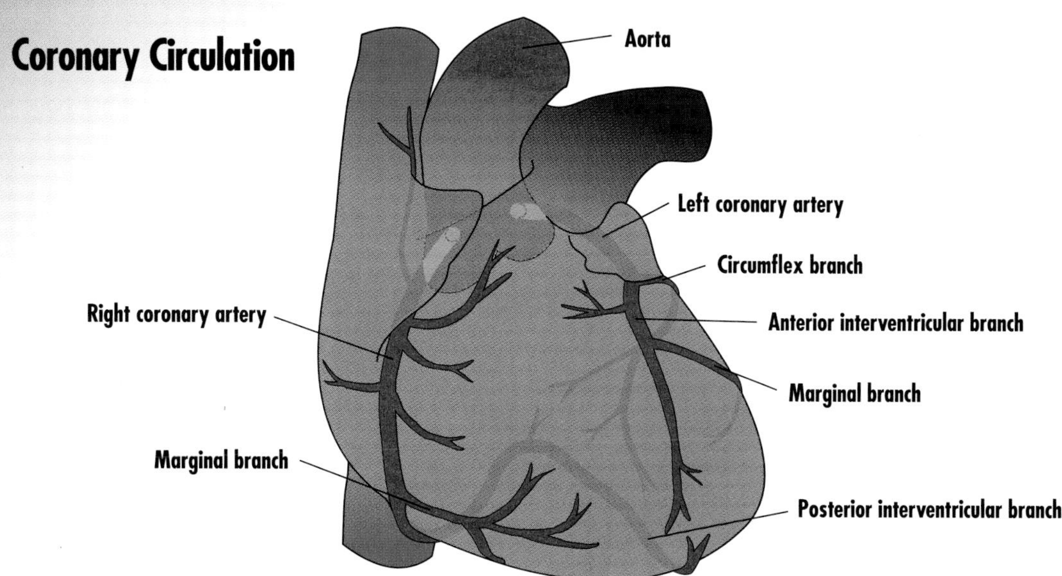

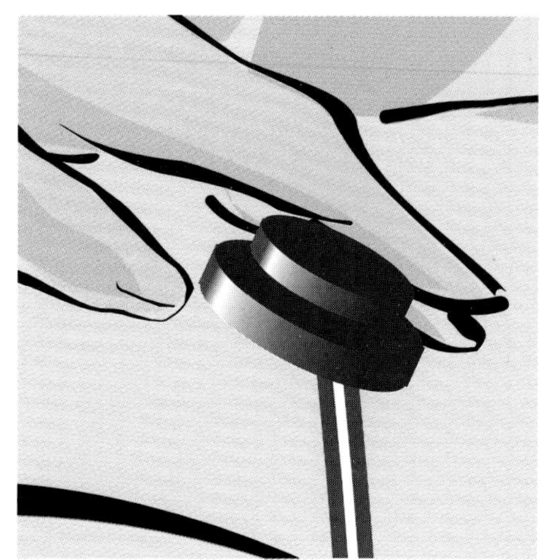

# How the Heart Beats

THE HEART HAS the unique ability to beat, or contract, on its own. Its normal functioning as a vital part of our bodies is assisted by nerves and hormones in the blood and, remarkably, it continues to function when removed from these influences. This unassisted functioning ability is best illustrated by the donor organ in heart transplantations.

The mechanism by which the heart generates and transmits the signal to contract is quite complex. Actually, minute electrical impulses are generated by a specialized group of cells in the wall of the right atrium, called the *sinoatrial (SA) node*, the heart's internal pacemaker. Each impulse passes down from its origin through the conducting system of the heart, causing muscular contraction of each chamber as it passes through it.

Leaving the SA node, the impulse passes through both atria, causing them to contract and helping blood to pass into their respective ventricles. On its way to the ventricles, the impulse next encounters the *atrioventricular (AV) node*, another group of specialized cells. From there, the impulse passes down an anatomic pathway called the *Bundle of His,* which divides into Left and Right Bundle Branches. The impulse moves through the Branches into the terminal Purkinje fibers, conduction pathways which distribute the stimulus to myocardial cells and cause the ventricles to contract.

The electrical process that accompanies contraction is called *depolarization*. During relaxation from the contraction, *repolarization* occurs and the contracting cells return to their original state. This complex series of events occurs in less than a second, with every beat of the heart.

The electrocardiogram (ECG) is a reflection of the electrical events that occur in the heart during each contraction. The electrocardiograph, the machine producing the ECG, is an essential tool of the physician for diagnosing and monitoring heart conditions. Taking an ECG is a simple and safe procedure and is an important part of a physical examination, especially when a heart problem is being considered. Many physicians require an ECG to be taken routinely as part of the examination of a person over 40 years old.

By means of electrodes placed on the chest, arms, and legs, the ECG records and amplifies the electrical events of the heart. A permanent record is available immediately for interpretation. The ECG helps the physician detect abnormalities in heart rhythm and rate as well as abnormalities associated with the myocardium, such as the presence of old or new myocardial infarctions. The ECG is also used in conjunction with other tests.

The deflections, or movements from the base line of the ECG have been given arbitrary designations. Each cardiac cycle begins with a P wave, representing contraction of the atria, which is followed by a short pause, the PR interval, while the impulse is traveling to the ventricles. Ventricular depolarization is represented by a complex series of waves designated as the QRS complex. The R wave is the most prominent component of this complex and represents the forceful ventricular contraction. The final wave of the ECG is the T wave, representing repolarization and a return to the resting state of the ventricles. The interval between the QRS complex and the T wave is called the ST segment.

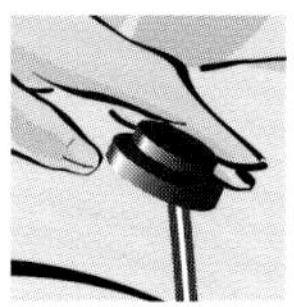

# How an Electrical Impulse Becomes a Heartbeat

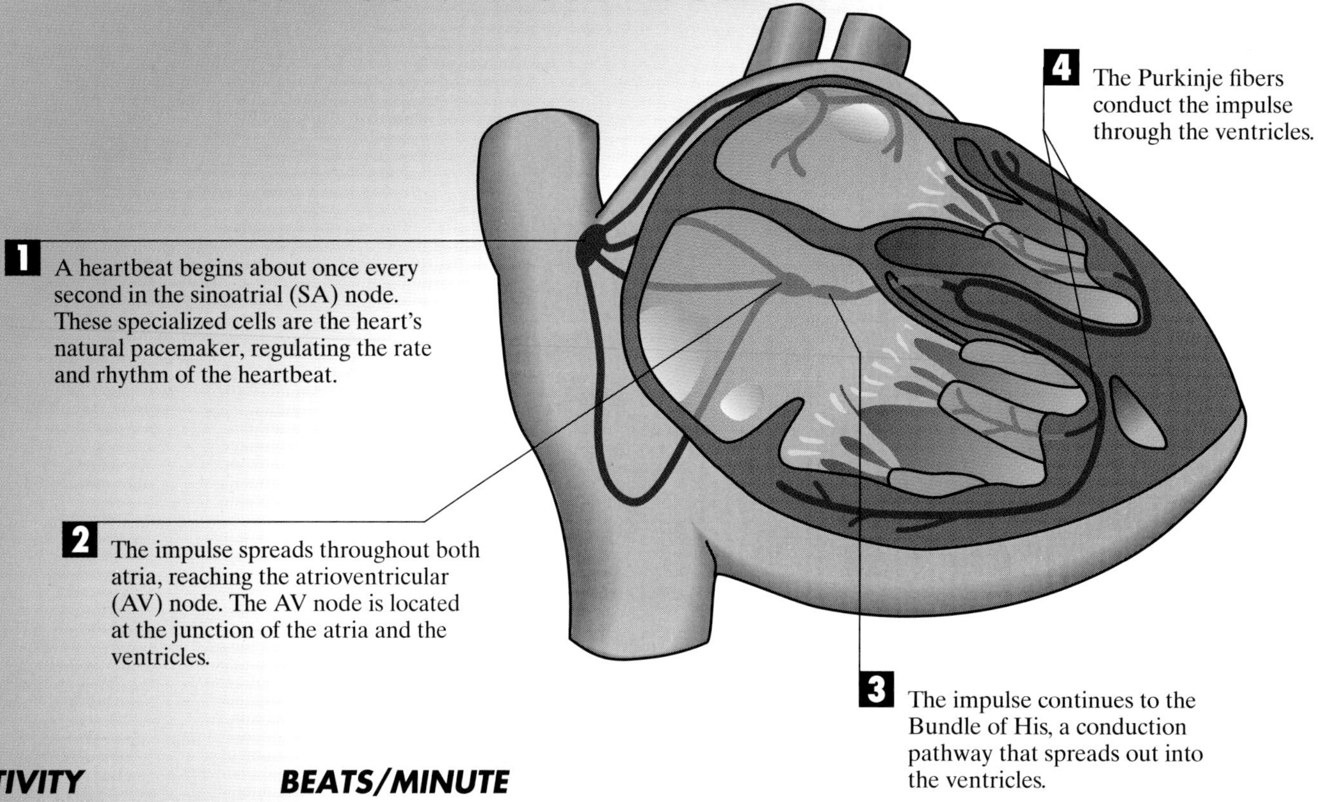

**1** A heartbeat begins about once every second in the sinoatrial (SA) node. These specialized cells are the heart's natural pacemaker, regulating the rate and rhythm of the heartbeat.

**2** The impulse spreads throughout both atria, reaching the atrioventricular (AV) node. The AV node is located at the junction of the atria and the ventricles.

**3** The impulse continues to the Bundle of His, a conduction pathway that spreads out into the ventricles.

**4** The Purkinje fibers conduct the impulse through the ventricles.

| *ACTIVITY* | *BEATS/MINUTE* |
|---|---|
| Sleeping | 60 – 70 |
| Walking | 80 – 100 |
| Riding a bike | 110 – 130 |
| After a meal | 80 – 90 |
| Watching an exciting sports event | 80 – 90 |
| Moderate fever | 90 |

## The Electrocardiogram of One Heartbeat

The electrocardiogram (ECG) is a simple and painless process requiring only a few minutes; it is a most valuable diagnostic and therapeutic tool. The ECG consists of a series of deflections and lines, each one representing a different component of the cardiac cycle, or heartbeat. Abnormalities in the ECG are valuable clues in the diagnosis of heart disease, and subsequent changes are important indicators of the progress of the disease.

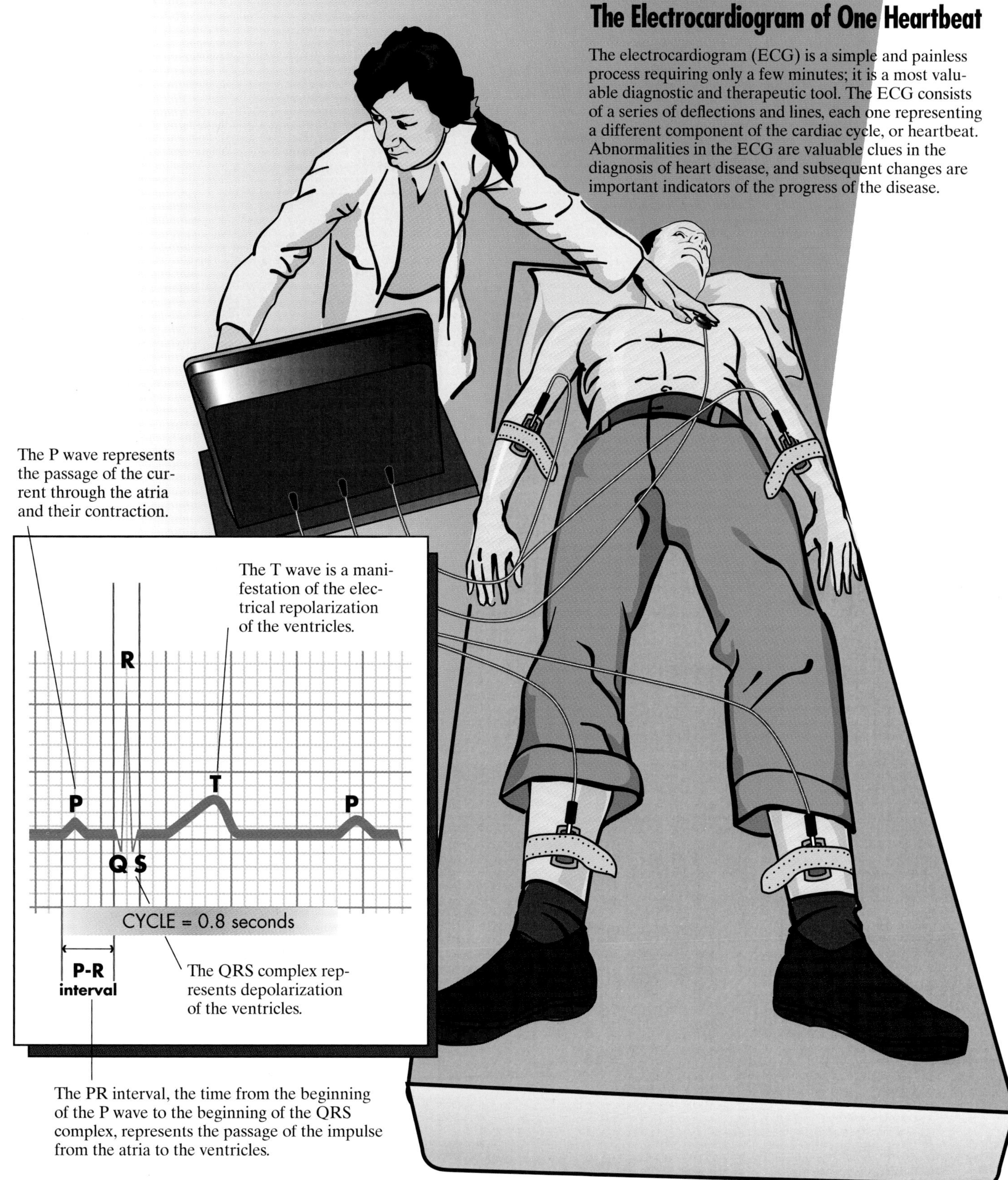


The P wave represents the passage of the current through the atria and their contraction.

The T wave is a manifestation of the electrical repolarization of the ventricles.

The QRS complex represents depolarization of the ventricles.

The PR interval, the time from the beginning of the P wave to the beginning of the QRS complex, represents the passage of the impulse from the atria to the ventricles.

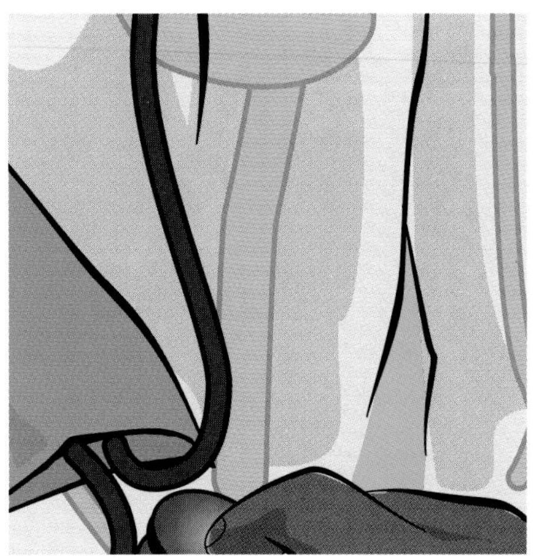

# Vital Signs

STARTING DURING FETAL life, the heart works ceaselessly, driving blood through the body's blood vessels. In a full lifetime, the heart will beat over 2 billion times, sending blood through 60,000 miles of blood vessels. The contractile, or ejection, phase of the cardiac cycle is referred to as *systole*; the relaxation phase, during which the chambers refill with blood, is referred to as *diastole*. The volume of blood pumped out of the heart during each left ventricular contraction is referred to as the *stroke volume*. Each contraction ejects a little over 2 ounces, which is about 10 pints per minute, or 2,500 to 3,000 gallons per day.

The term *cardiac output* refers to the amount of blood that the heart pumps per minute and can be derived from the formula *cardiac output equals stroke volume times heart rate per minute*. It has been well demonstrated that stroke volume changes very little under normal circumstances. The exception to this rule is in well-trained athletes who are capable of increasing stroke volume. For most of us, changes in cardiac output are related to changes in the heart rate. As the heart rate increases, cardiac output is increased, and as the heart rate decreases, cardiac output decreases. The normal heart rate varies between 60 and 100 beats per minute, but is usually around 72 beats per minute. A heart rate slower than 60 beats per minute is referred to as *bradycardia* (brady means slow), and a heart rate in excess of 100 beats per minute is referred to as *tachycardia* (tachy means rapid). Thus, when an increase in cardiac output is required in such instances as stress, excitement, exercise, and fever, the sympathetic nervous system causes an increase in pulse rate while stroke volume remains unchanged.

Left ventricular contraction produces a surge of blood through the blood vessels that gives rise to two important vital signs. Vital signs are readily available indices used to monitor the general state of health of an individual and include pulse, blood pressure, body temperature, and rate of breathing or respiration. In hospitalized patients, vital signs are the measurements the physician or nurse records on the patient's chart that provide an indication of the patient's general condition.

There are two vital signs that are generated by left ventricular contraction: pulse and blood pressure. The pulse is a direct result of the surge of blood produced by left ventricular contraction. It is a ready means of recognizing the rate and the regularity of the heartbeat. The strength of the pulse is also important; a weak, thready pulse may be an indication of a serious problem. The pulse can be taken at any point on the body surface where a large artery runs close to the skin. Common pulse sites are the neck, armpit, groin, and foot. For convenience, the pulse is usually taken at the wrist, near the base of the thumb, where the large radial artery to the hand is close to the skin. In case of doubt, the pulse can be verified by listening to the heart with a stethoscope, a procedure referred to as *auscultation*.

We will discuss changes in heart rate and regularity in greater detail in a subsequent chapter, and will illustrate these changes with electrocardiograms.

The blood pressure, the second of the vital signs related to the heart, consists of two components: the *systolic* and the *diastolic* blood pressures. The systolic blood pressure is the pressure generated by left ventricular contraction and assisted by arterial compression. The diastolic pressure is the residual pressure in the arterial system during the dilation phase of ventricular relaxation and refilling. It is important to remember that there is always a supply of blood in the vascular system during both of these phases.

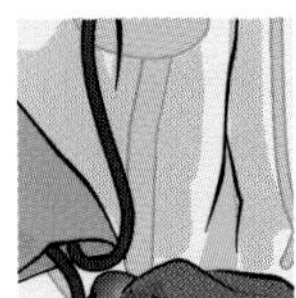

Blood pressure is measured by various types of *sphygmomanometers*, which register the pressure in terms of the height of a column of mercury expressed in millimeters. (Mercury, a liquid element 13 times heavier than water, provides an easy and useful means of measurement. If we had to use water, for example, the column would be far too high to handle.) The blood pressure is expressed as the ratio of systolic/diastolic pressures. Normally, the systolic pressure is 140 millimeters of mercury (mm Hg) or less, and the diastolic pressure is 90 mm Hg or less at rest. *Hypertension* (high blood pressure) exists when either the systolic or diastolic readings are repeatedly above 140 and 90 mm Hg, respectively. We will discuss hypertension in greater detail in a subsequent chapter.

There are no set standards for *hypotension* (low blood pressure) because it is relative to the patient's known normal blood pressure. Thus, a systolic blood pressure of 120 mm Hg, considered normal under usual conditions, might represent hypotension in an individual who previously had a systolic blood pressure of 180 mm Hg. Generally speaking, however, a systolic blood pressure of 100 mm Hg or below suggests hypotension. The diagnosis is usually made in the presence of other confirmatory signs and symptoms.

# Vital Signs

## Taking the Blood Pressure

The physician takes a patient's blood pressure using a mercury sphygmomanometer. By compressing the bulb, the cuff around the arm is inflated and the column of mercury rises. Blood pressure has two components, the systolic and diastolic blood pressures, which are recorded as a ratio or fraction. Systolic blood pressure measures the force created by left ventricular contraction and assisted by arterial compression. The diastolic pressure measures the residual pressure in the arterial system when the ventricle is dilating, or relaxing and filling with blood. Normal blood pressure has a systolic measurement of 140 mm Hg and a diastolic measurement of 90 mm Hg or less. This is commonly stated as 140/90 or 140 over 90. Repeated higher readings of one or both of the pressures is considered hypertension (high blood pressure).

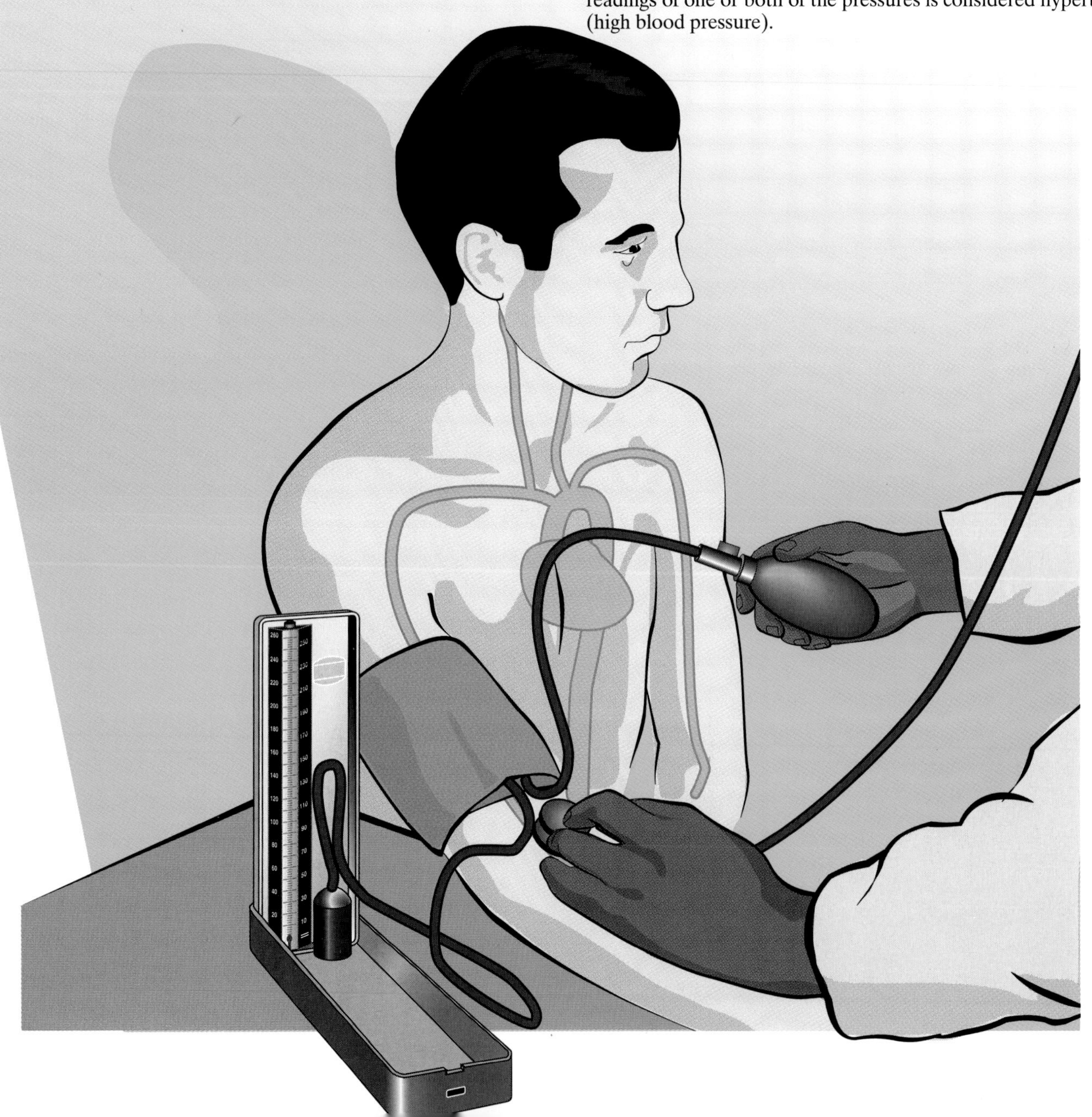

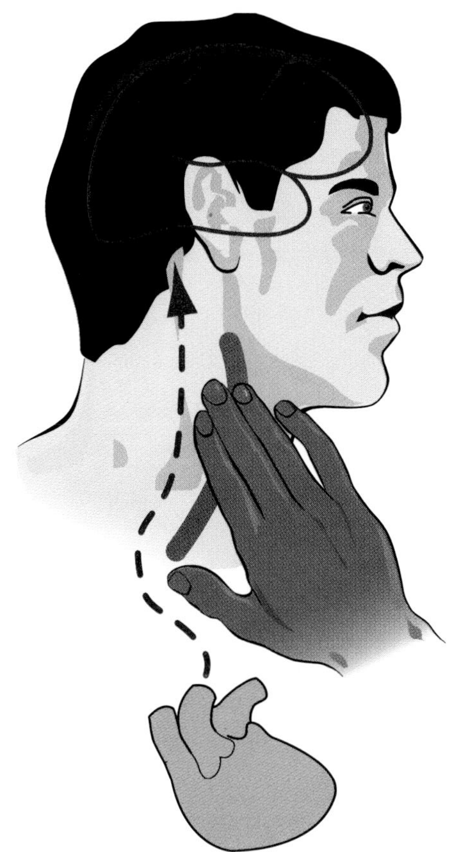

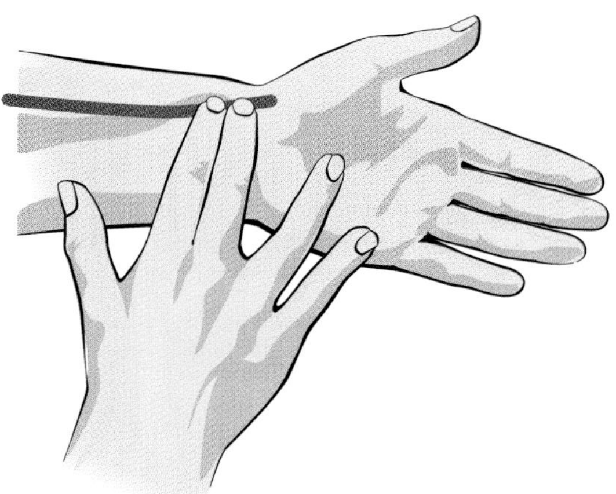

## Taking the Pulse

The pulse may be taken at any place where a large artery is close to the surface of the skin. The illustration shows the pulse being taken in the neck where the large carotid artery passes, and branches to the neck, face, tongue, and palate, and eventually reaches the brain. The carotid pulse may be felt to the left or right of the larynx (Adam's apple). Both arteries should not be felt simultaneously because that may cause slowing of the heart and impairment of the circulation to the brain. The normal pulse rate in adults is about 72 beats per minute, but may vary between 60 and 100 beats per minute.

**Cardiac Output per Minute=Stroke Volume per Beat × Pulse Rate per Minute** The blood output of the heart per minute can be calculated by the simple formula above. Inasmuch as the stroke volume per beat remains relatively constant in most of us, the pulse rate is the important determinate of cardiac output. When it increases because of exercise, excitement, and other emotions, cardiac output increases. If the pulse rate slows, cardiac output decreases.

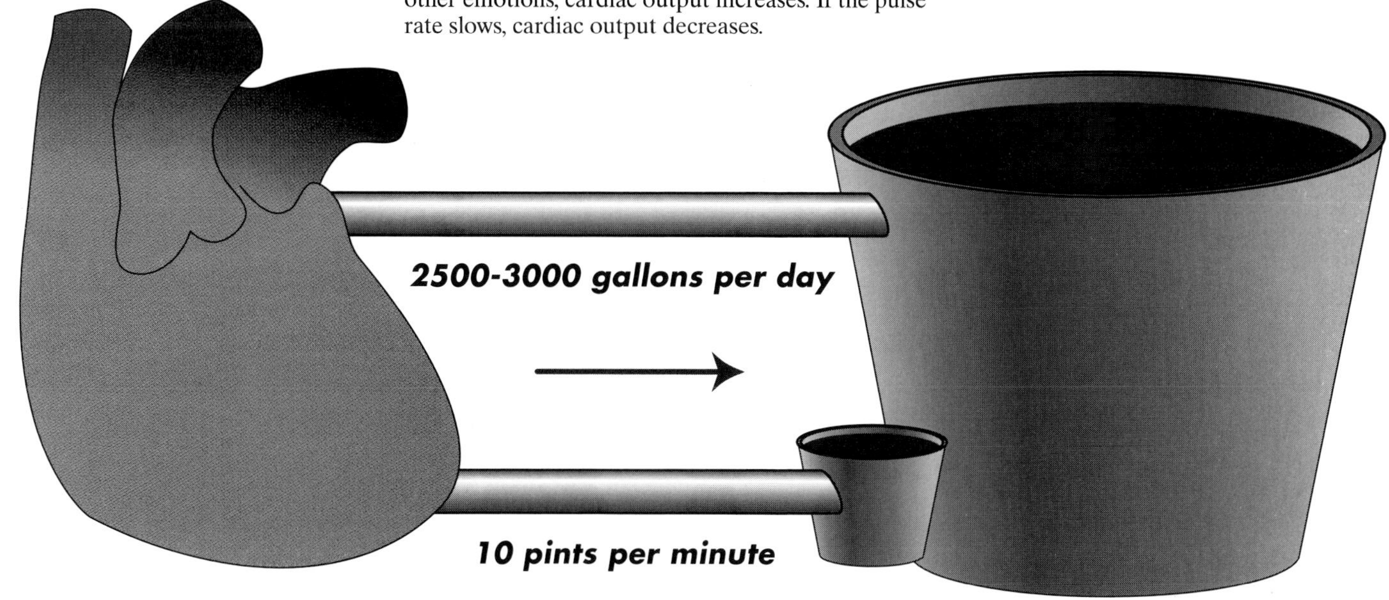

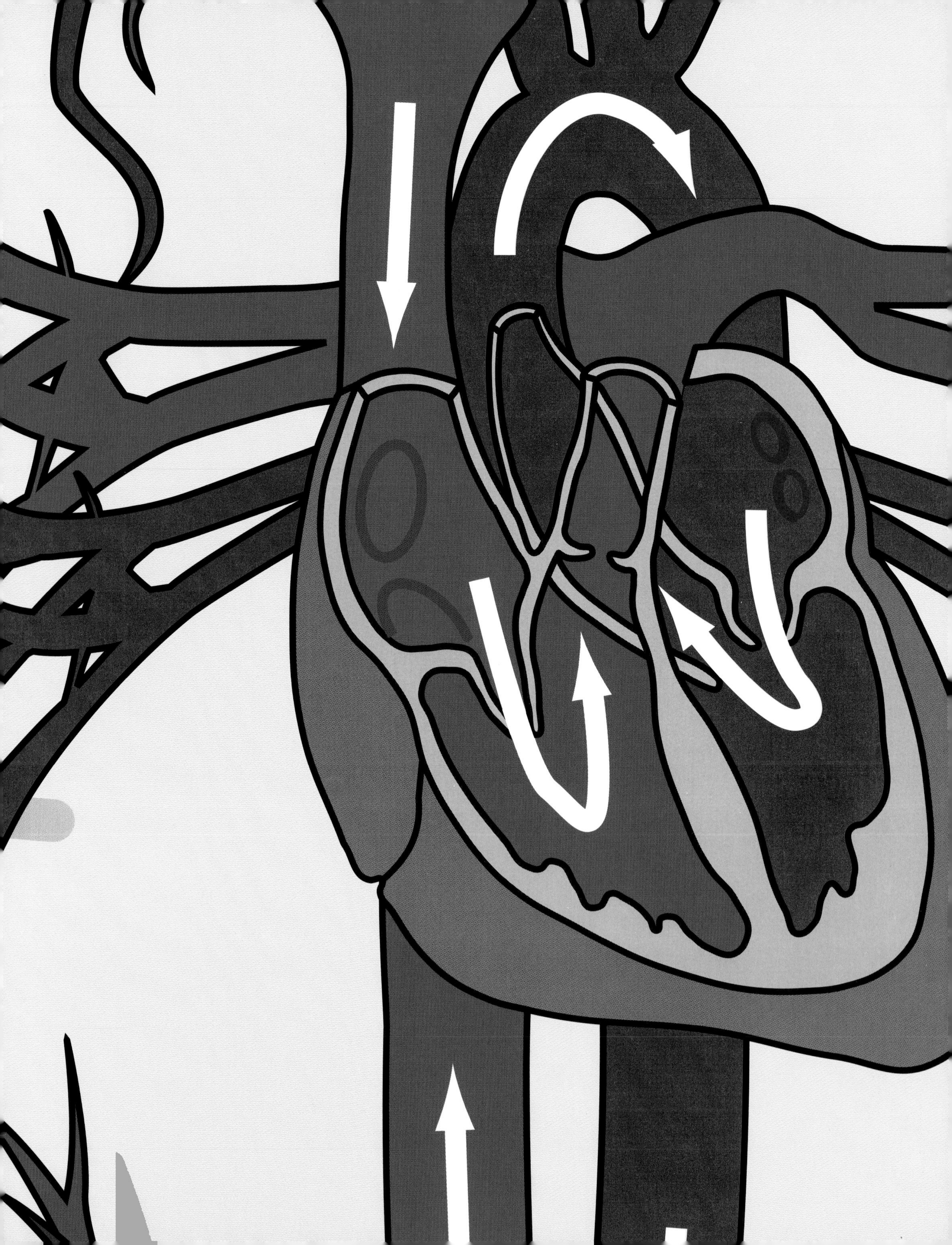

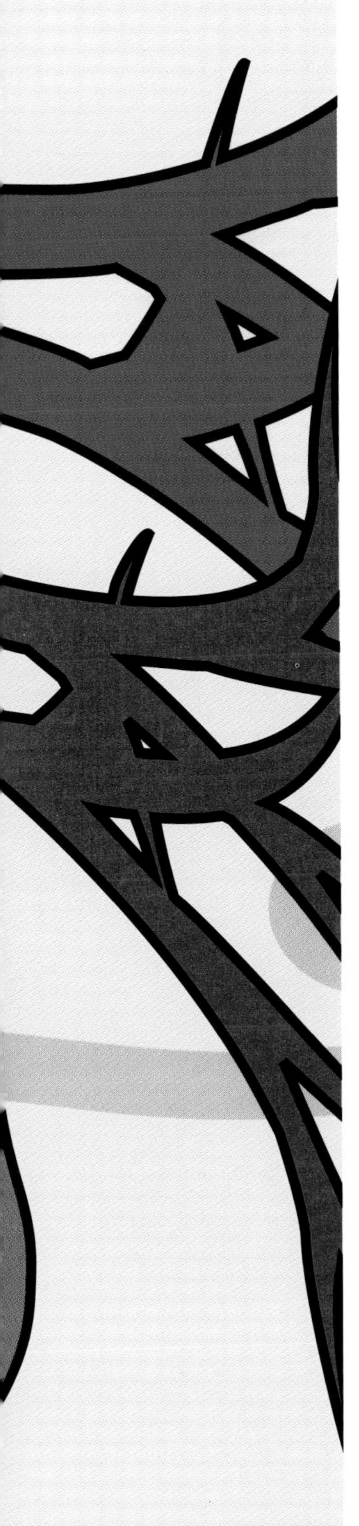

# 2 THE NORMAL VASCULAR SYSTEM

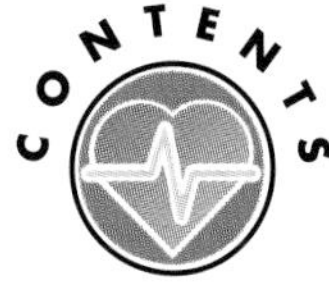

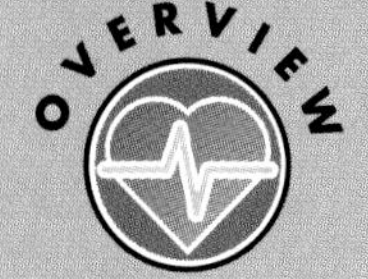
OVERVIEW

THE BLOOD PUMPED by the heart is distributed by a complex 60,000-mile network of blood vessels—the vascular system (the word *vascular* is derived from the Latin words for canal or vessel, *vas* or *vasculum*).

The vascular system is divided into three components. The *arterial system* is responsible for the delivery of blood and oxygen to every cell, tissue, and organ in the body. The arteries carry blood away from the heart. Veins comprise the *venous system* that is responsible for returning deoxygenated (deprived of oxygen) blood from the tissues and organs back to the heart. The *capillary system* (from the Latin, *capillaria*, for thread) is responsible for the exchange of oxygen for carbon dioxide at the cellular level.

As you will see in Chapters 4, 5, and 6, the vascular system is not a passive system of pipes, but actually plays an important active role in supplementing the action of the heart in the distribution of blood.

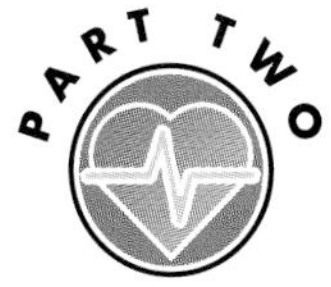

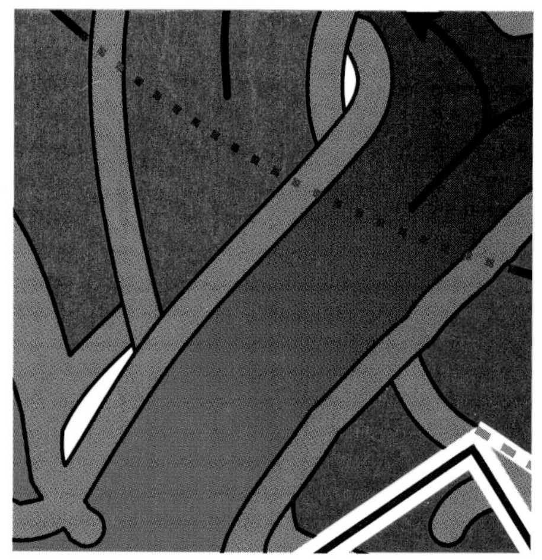

# The Arterial System

THE ARTERIAL SYSTEM is responsible for the transportation of blood from the heart to the cells, tissues, and organs. During left ventricular *systole,* or contraction, blood leaves the heart by way of the *aorta*, the largest blood vessel in the body. The *aortic valve* is situated at the entrance to the aorta. When the left ventricle contracts, the valve opens, allowing, under normal circumstances, the free flow of blood into the aorta. *Diastole* is the relaxation and refilling portion of the cardiac cycle. During this phase, the aortic valve closes, preventing regurgitation of blood from the aorta back into the left ventricle. Anatomically, the aortic valve consists of three cusps (posterior, right, and left) that come together during diastole to completely occlude the valve and prevent regurgitation. Because the edge of each cusp is in the shape of a half moon, the valve is also called the *semilunar* valve.

Within the left and right cusps of the aortic valve are the left and right coronary arteries, which form the coronary circulation and provide oxygenated blood to the heart muscle itself. From the arch of the aorta, two large branches, called the carotid arteries, go into either side of the neck, supplying blood to the neck and most of the brain. The carotid arteries are the ones whose pulses you can feel in your neck. Large branches from the aorta are also sent to supply blood to the arms. Then the aorta passes down the back of the body in front of the spine supplying branches to the internal organs. The last large branches of the aorta go to the legs.

As the arteries approach their destination, they become increasingly smaller and are called *arterioles*. Finally, they reach their smallest size, having a threadlike diameter, and are called *capillaries*.

The arteries play an important role in supplementing the heart's action in the circulation of the blood. If you examine the wall of an artery under a microscope, several layers are apparent. The *endothelium* or *intima*, the delicate inner lining of the blood vessel, may become damaged with *arteriosclerosis*, commonly referred to as hardening of the arteries. We will discuss arteriosclerosis and the role of cholesterol in its formation later in the book. The aorta and other large vessels also have a layer of elastic tissue, which stretches to accommodate the blood pumped during systole, and then recoils to propel the blood forward. Arteries also have a layer of smooth muscle, which is capable of decreasing and increasing the diameter of the blood vessel. This is how the artery is able to control the amount of blood passing through it.

*Vasoconstriction* is the constriction or narrowing of an artery, which raises blood pressure. Vasoconstrictors are formed within the body, especially in the adrenal glands and kidneys. There are medications with vasoconstriction action that are helpful in the control of bleeding.

*Vasodilation,* or dilation of the blood vessels, occurs in the body under certain circumstances and results in a decrease in blood pressure, as in shock, for example. There are medications that have vasodilator properties and these drugs are important in the treatment of hypertension. They may also be used to increase the blood supply to areas where the arterial circulation has been compromised, including the coronary circulation. Both vasoconstriction and vasodilation are controlled by hormones and nerves in our bodies, over which we have little or no voluntary control.

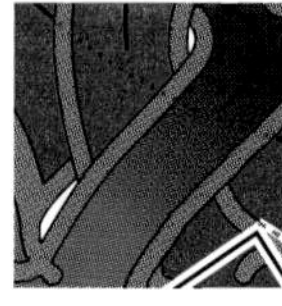

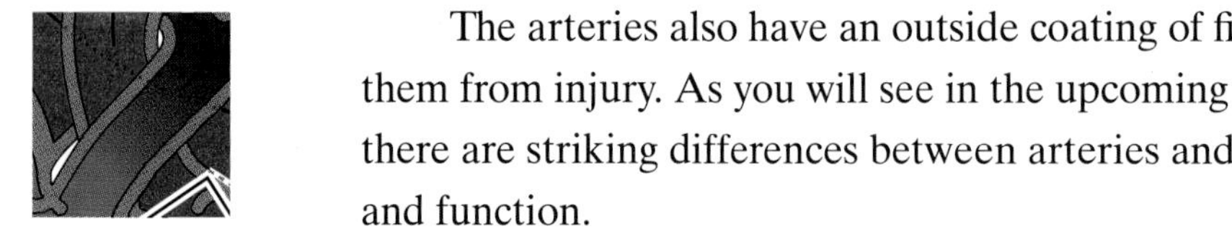

The arteries also have an outside coating of fibrous tissue that helps to protect them from injury. As you will see in the upcoming discussions on the venous system, there are striking differences between arteries and veins in their structure, physiology, and function.

# The Arterial System

## The Arterial Tree

The arterial system is responsible for the transport of oxygenated blood from the heart to all the cells, tissues, and organs of the body. As the large artery (the *aorta*) leaves the heart, it curves to the left, forming an arch. The main blood vessels to the neck, head, and arms emanate from the arch of the aorta. The aorta then courses downward behind the heart and in front of the spine. As it descends, it issues numerous branches to the chest and to the organs of the abdomen. Finally, as it reaches the pelvis, the aorta divides into two large branches (*bifurcation of the aorta*), each large branch supplying one of the lower extremities. Secondary and tertiary smaller arteries are called *arterioles*. Eventually, within the substance of the tissues and organs, the arterioles become threadlike, forming the arterial side of the *capillary system*.

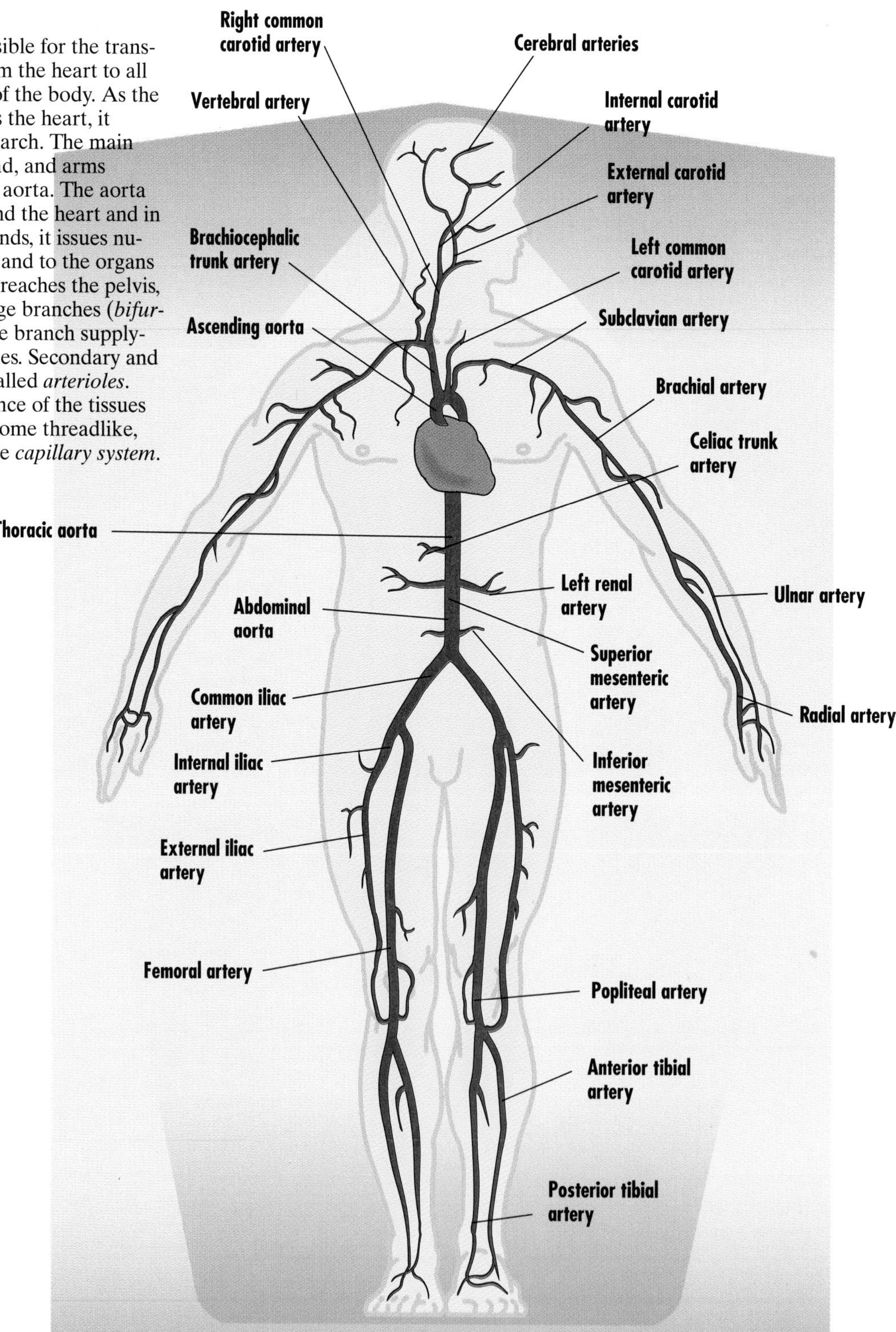

## Arterial Blood Flow to and from the Heart

We have already discussed the flow of arterial blood from the heart. Of equal importance is the supply of arterial blood to the heart. The heart receives its supply of oxygenated blood from the lungs by way of the *pulmonary veins*. These important vessels deliver their cargo to the left atrium and thence to the left ventricle by way of the *mitral* or *bicuspid* valve, which lies between the left atrium and the left ventricle. Disease of the mitral valve may interfere with this process and have serious effects on the heart and circulation.

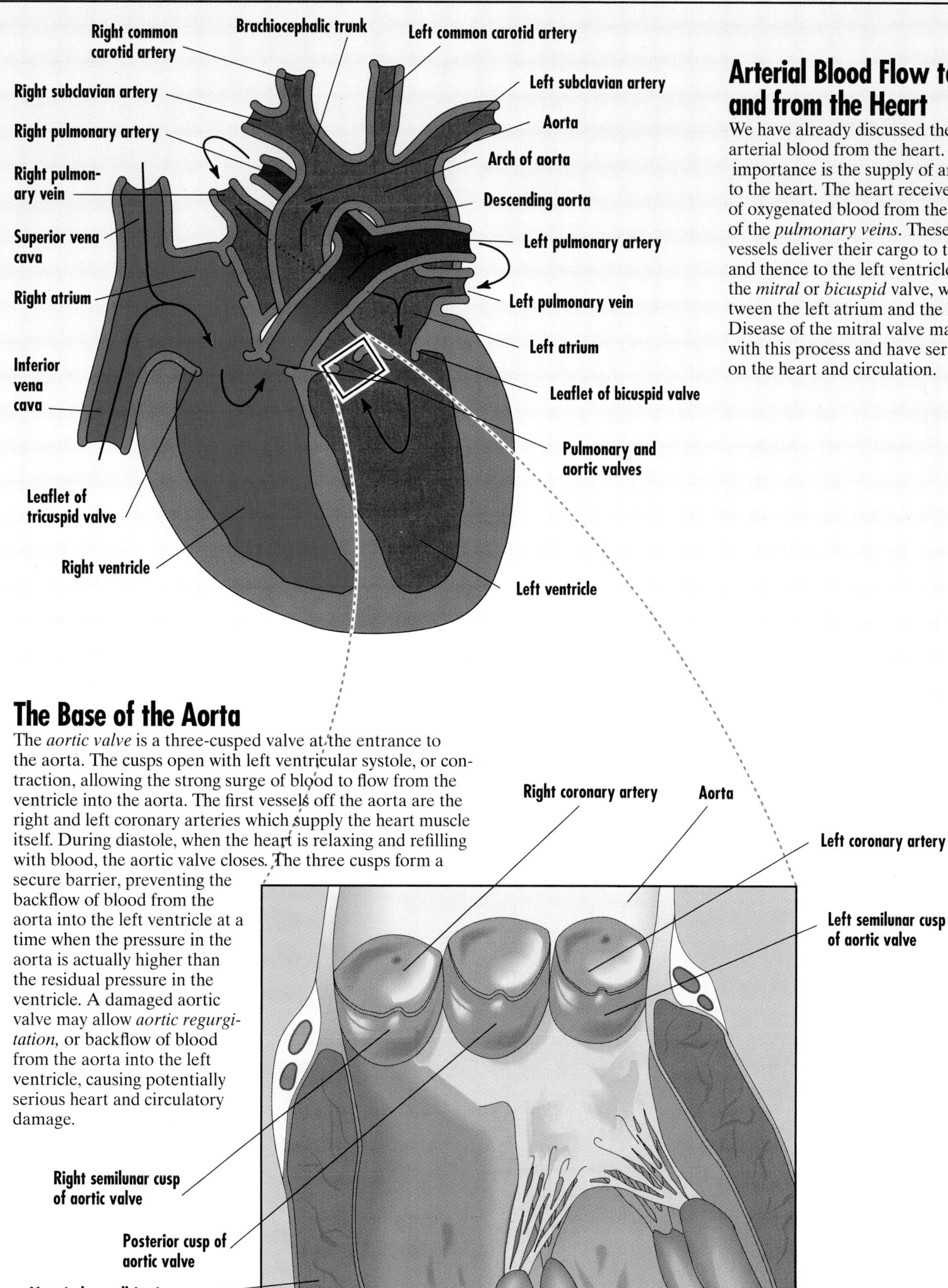


## The Base of the Aorta

The *aortic valve* is a three-cusped valve at the entrance to the aorta. The cusps open with left ventricular systole, or contraction, allowing the strong surge of blood to flow from the ventricle into the aorta. The first vessels off the aorta are the right and left coronary arteries which supply the heart muscle itself. During diastole, when the heart is relaxing and refilling with blood, the aortic valve closes. The three cusps form a secure barrier, preventing the backflow of blood from the aorta into the left ventricle at a time when the pressure in the aorta is actually higher than the residual pressure in the ventricle. A damaged aortic valve may allow *aortic regurgitation,* or backflow of blood from the aorta into the left ventricle, causing potentially serious heart and circulatory damage.

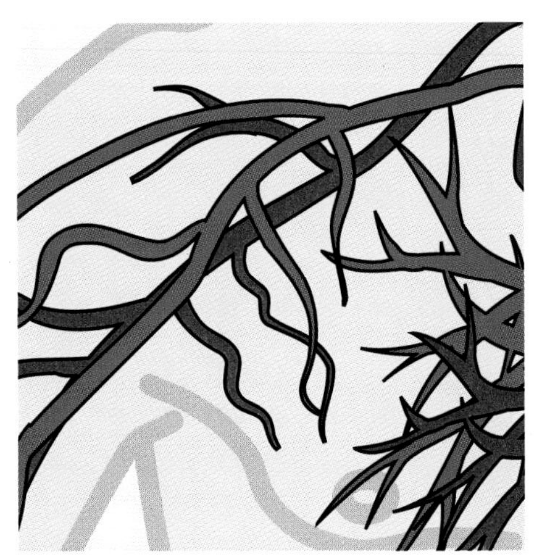

# The Venous System

JUST AS THE arteries take blood away from the heart, veins are responsible for the return of blood from the tissues and organs of the body to the heart. The blood carried by the venous system has been depleted of oxygen ($O_2$) in exchange for carbon dioxide ($CO_2$). The transport of the blood from the heart to the lungs for replenishment of oxygen is considered to be part of the venous system.

Because blood is constantly flowing to and from the heart, arteries and veins branch throughout the body in a parallel system, for the most part. This system may be likened to a divided highway: Imagine a road with traffic on either side flowing in opposite directions. The blood flows throughout the body in similar, parallel, but opposite sytems, with one system of "traffic" traveling at a faster pace than the other. In many instances, arteries and veins share the same name. All venous channels from the head and chest lead into the *superior vena cava.* Blood from below the chest drains into the *inferior vena cava.* Both of these large veins empty into the right atrium, from which their contents are passed into the right ventricle. Right ventricular contraction then pumps the blood to the lungs by way of the *pulmonary arteries.*

There are striking anatomical and physiological differences between arteries and veins. Whereas arteries are strong, muscular, and elastic, veins are more delicate in structure and, to a significant degree, lack the elasticity and muscular power of the arteries. Veins have a limited capability for vasoconstriction, but have a large capacity for vasodilation. Arterial blood flow is much faster than venous blood flow because it reflects the power of the left ventricular contraction as well as the artery's own capability for contraction. Arterial bleeding is pulsatile, again reflecting the contraction of the left ventricle; venous bleeding is slower and more steady in character. In some of the major arteries, blood moves at a rate of over 1 foot per second, whereas the flow rate in veins is about 4 inches per second. The venous pressure varies throughout the body, depending on the position of the individual and the site of measurement. Venous pressure averages 50 to 100 mm of water, much lower than the pressure of 120 mm of the much heavier mercury seen in arteries during contraction. (Since venous pressure is much lower than arterial pressure, it is measured by using a column of water rather than the much heavier mercury that we use for arterial blood pressure.) Arterial blood is much brighter and redder than venous blood because of its oxygen content.

Veins have valves that prevent the reversal of the flow of venous blood. For example, standing upright for a prolonged period would be expected to increase the venous pressure in the legs and promote the backflow of blood. Pressure does increase, but venous valves prevent the reversal of blood. Unfortunately, the valves are prone to damage and this may result in *edema* or swelling and the presence of permanently dilated veins (*varicose veins*).

The veins have a greater capacity to widen or dilate than do arteries. Because of this, the volume of blood in our venous system is 2 to 2½ times that of the arterial system. This pool of blood acts as an important reservoir that becomes available if the circumstances require more blood, such as occurs in shock, serious injuries, severe bleeding, or anything that results in a sudden drop in blood presure. Changes in the venous circulation that make more blood available for increased cardiac output are vital in these conditions. Thus, the venous circulation, once thought to play a rather passive role in the circulation and serve only as a passageway for the flow of blood, is now recognized as playing an important active role in circulation.

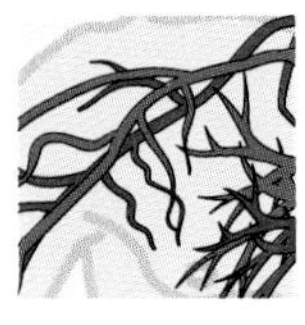

# The Venous System

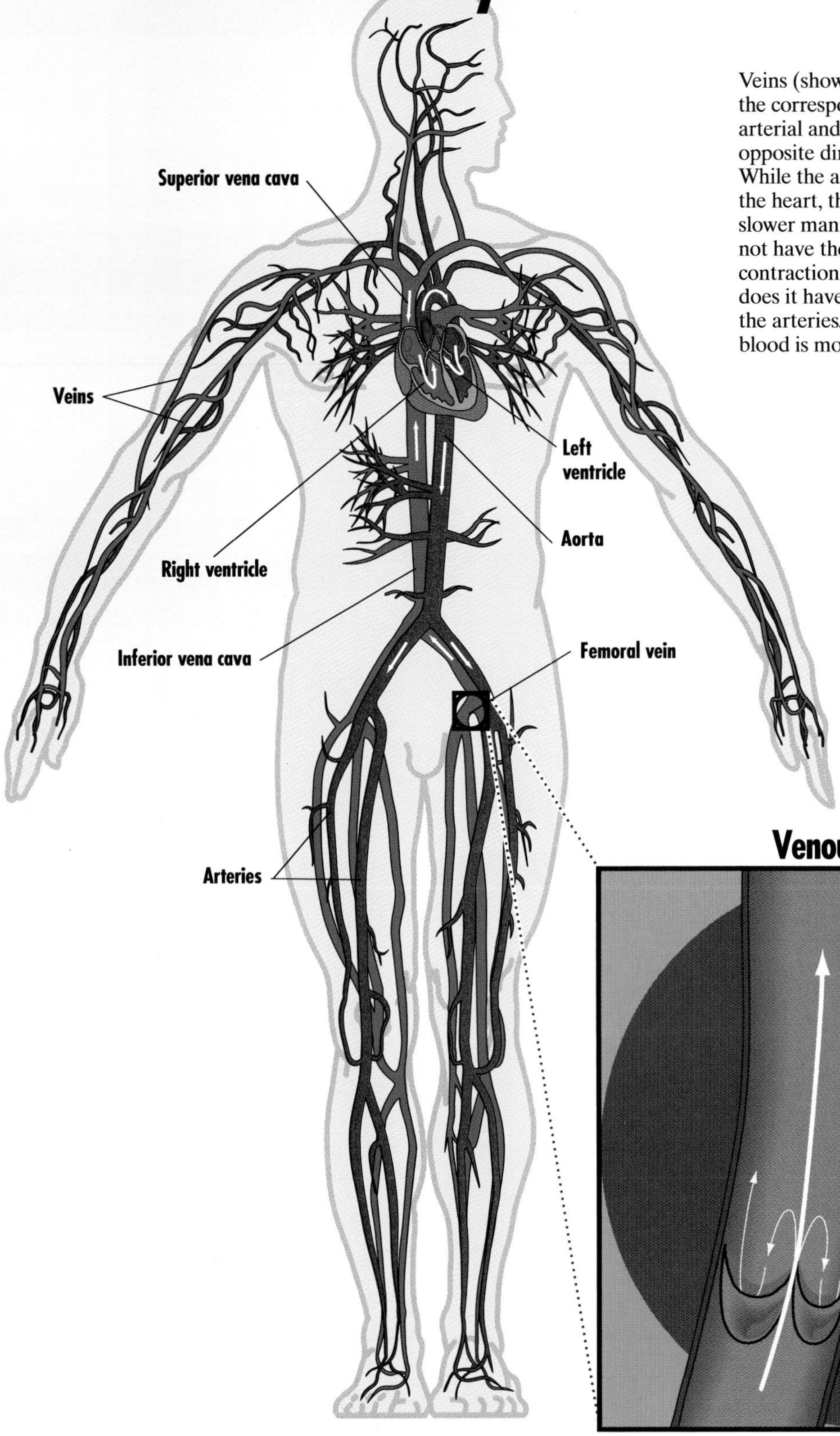

Superior vena cava

Veins

Right ventricle

Inferior vena cava

Arteries

Left ventricle

Aorta

Femoral vein

Veins (shown in blue) are generally parallel to the corresponding arteries (shown in red). The arterial and venous blood, however, flows in opposite directions and at different speeds: While the arteries swiftly take blood away from the heart, the veins return blood to the heart in a slower manner because venous blood flow does not have the impetus provided by ventricular contraction that the arterial system has, nor does it have the intrinsic propulsive power of the arteries. As a result, the volume of venous blood is more than twice that of arterial blood.

Veins possess valves that prevent the slower-moving, larger-volume venous blood from pooling in the lower extremities when an individual has been in the upright position for a long time. The valves act like pockets to prevent the blood from flowing in a reverse direction.

## Venous Valves

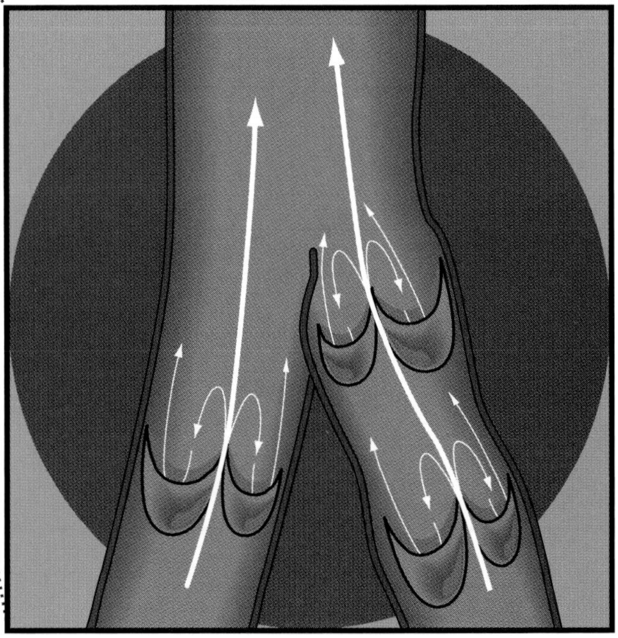

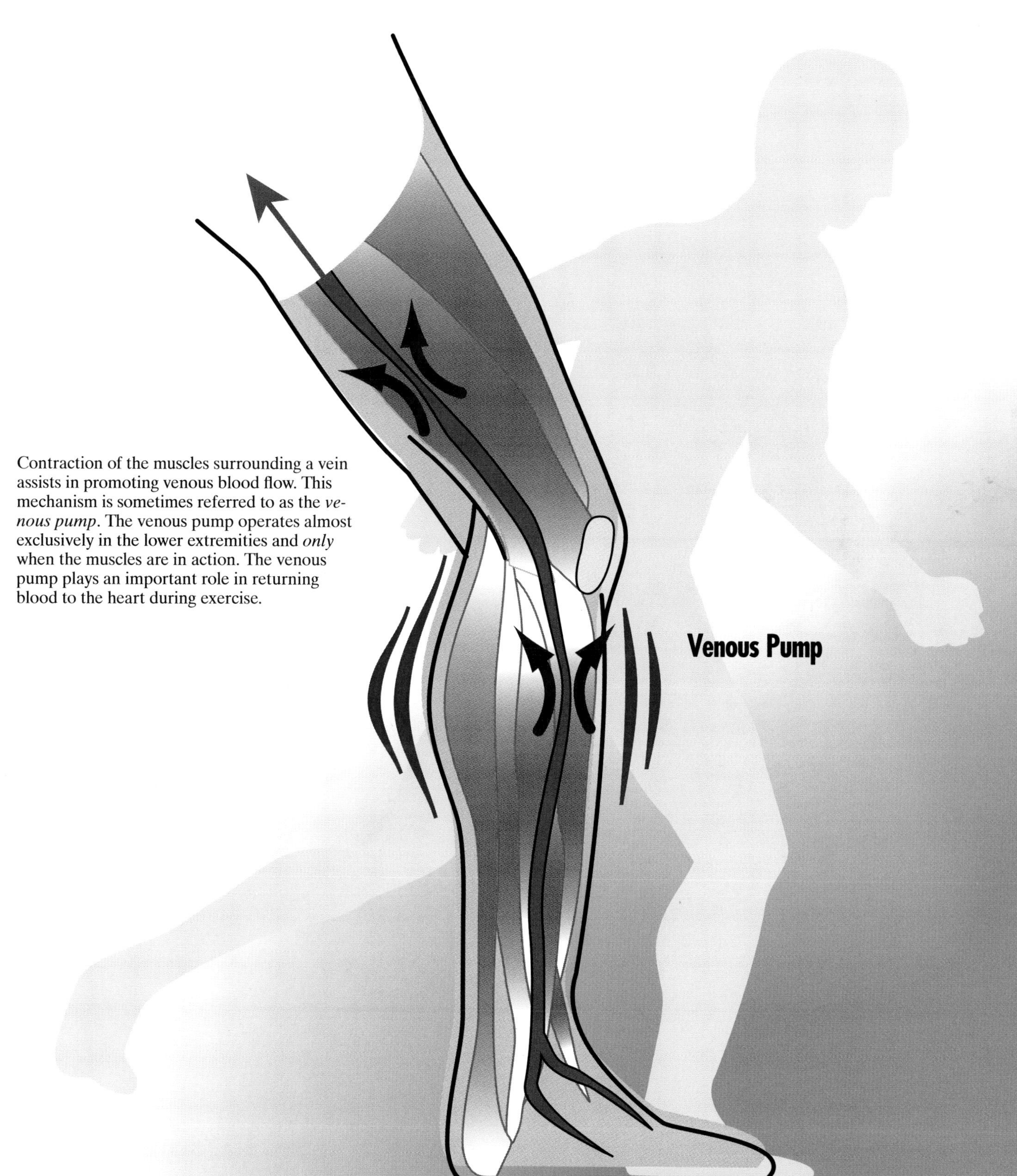


Contraction of the muscles surrounding a vein assists in promoting venous blood flow. This mechanism is sometimes referred to as the *venous pump*. The venous pump operates almost exclusively in the lower extremities and *only* when the muscles are in action. The venous pump plays an important role in returning blood to the heart during exercise.

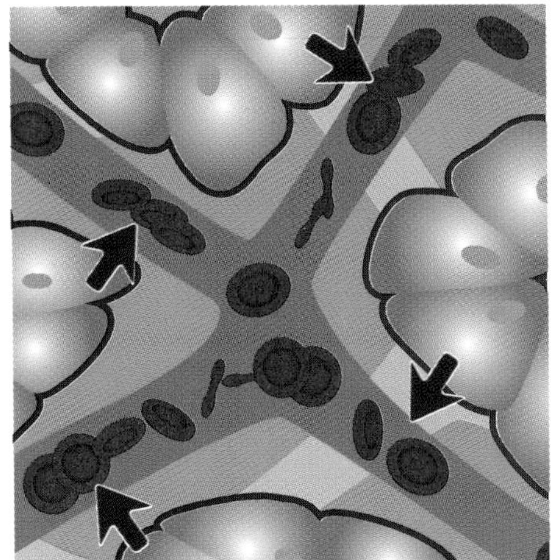

# The Capillary System

NOW THAT WE have examined the route of the blood to and from the heart by way of the venous and arterial systems, let's examine the process of exchange of substances that occurs between the blood and every tissue and organ in the body. This process is called an "exchange" because transfer of substances occurs in both directions, from blood to tissue and organs and vice versa. Incidentally, we do differentiate organs from tissues. An organ is composed of several basic types of tissues working together to perform one or more functions. For example, the stomach is an organ composed of glandular, muscular, and connective tissue, with each type of tissue contributing to the functions of the whole organ.

It is the function of the *capillaries*, the threadlike blood vessels that link the arterial with the venous system, to exchange fluid, oxygen, carbon dioxide, nutrients, electrolytes, hormones, and other substances between the blood and the *interstitial space*—the space outside the capillaries and separating the cells. In the lungs, for example, the capillaries form a meshwork around the *alveoli*, the tiny air sacs of the lungs. This system maximizes gas exchange of oxygen and carbon dioxide.

The capillary walls are very thin, consisting of a single layer of cells, to allow the passage of small molecular-sized substances. This passage is done through tiny *pores* or *clefts* in the capillary wall. In addition, substances can be transported through the wall with the help of small bubbles called *vesicles,* which carry the substances within them. However, *diffusion* is the most important means by which substances are transferred from the *plasma,* the liquid portion of the blood, to the interstitial fluid surrounding the cells. Diffusion allows the passage of substances through the capillary wall without the necessity of pores, clefts, or vesicles. We will learn that diffusion occurs from an area of high concentration to an area of low concentration. The method of transportation that is used depends on many complex factors including the size of the particle, pressure and concentration differences between the capillary and the interstitial fluid, and the solubility of the substance in water and lipids (fats).

The body's most essential task is the continuous transport of oxygen from the blood to the tissues and the return of oxygen to the blood in exchange for carbon dioxide ($CO_2$). This is the exchange process that occurs in the pulmonary or lung-related capillary circulation. In the lungs, the capillary system takes up oxygen from the air sacs and gives up carbon dioxide to be exhaled.

The blood has special carriers for the oxygen that it delivers to the tissues; they are the *red blood cells*, tiny concave disks. Red blood cells are so small that about 75 billion of them would fit into a 1-inch cube. Red cells get their color from hemoglobin, a protein that contains iron and is capable of carrying, releasing, and retrieving oxygen.

In the tissues, oxygen leaves the blood for the interstitial fluid by the process of diffusion. The concentration or partial pressure of oxygen in the interstitial fluid is low because it has been used by the cells. On the other hand, the content of oxygen in the capillary is high. By the process of diffusion, oxygen passes from the area of high concentration to the area of low concentration. At the same time that oxygen is being distributed from the blood to the interstitial fluid, carbon dioxide, a waste product of the cells, is picked up by the blood and carried by way of the venous circulation to the right atrium and right ventricle and pumped to the lungs.

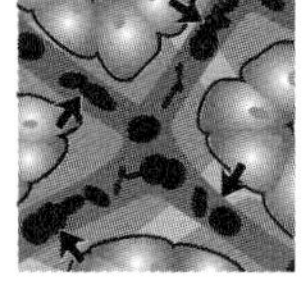

The exchange of carbon dioxide for oxygen occurs between the pulmonary capillary system and the alveoli, the tiny air sacs in the lungs that receive oxygen from inhaled air. The process again is one of diffusion across the delicate membrane that separates the blood in the pulmonary capillaries from the air in the alveoli.

These processes of gas—oxygen and carbon dioxide—exchange are continuous and essential for survival. Impairment of the process in tissue, lung, or blood by any mechanism may have serious consequences. The body does not tolerate low concentrations of oxygen and high concentrations of carbon dioxide for a prolonged period of time.

# The Capillary System

The capillary system is the link between the arterial and the venous systems. After the exchange of oxygen and carbon dioxide that occurs at the tissue level, the deoxygenated blood returns to the heart and is pumped by the right ventricle to the lungs, where oxygen is restored in place of carbon dioxide. As oxygen is given up in the tissues, the blood changes color, turning from a brilliant red to a dusky reddish-blue color. The figure greatly magnifies the size of the capillaries. Actually, at the tissue level, the capillaries are so tiny that they can only be seen under a microscope.

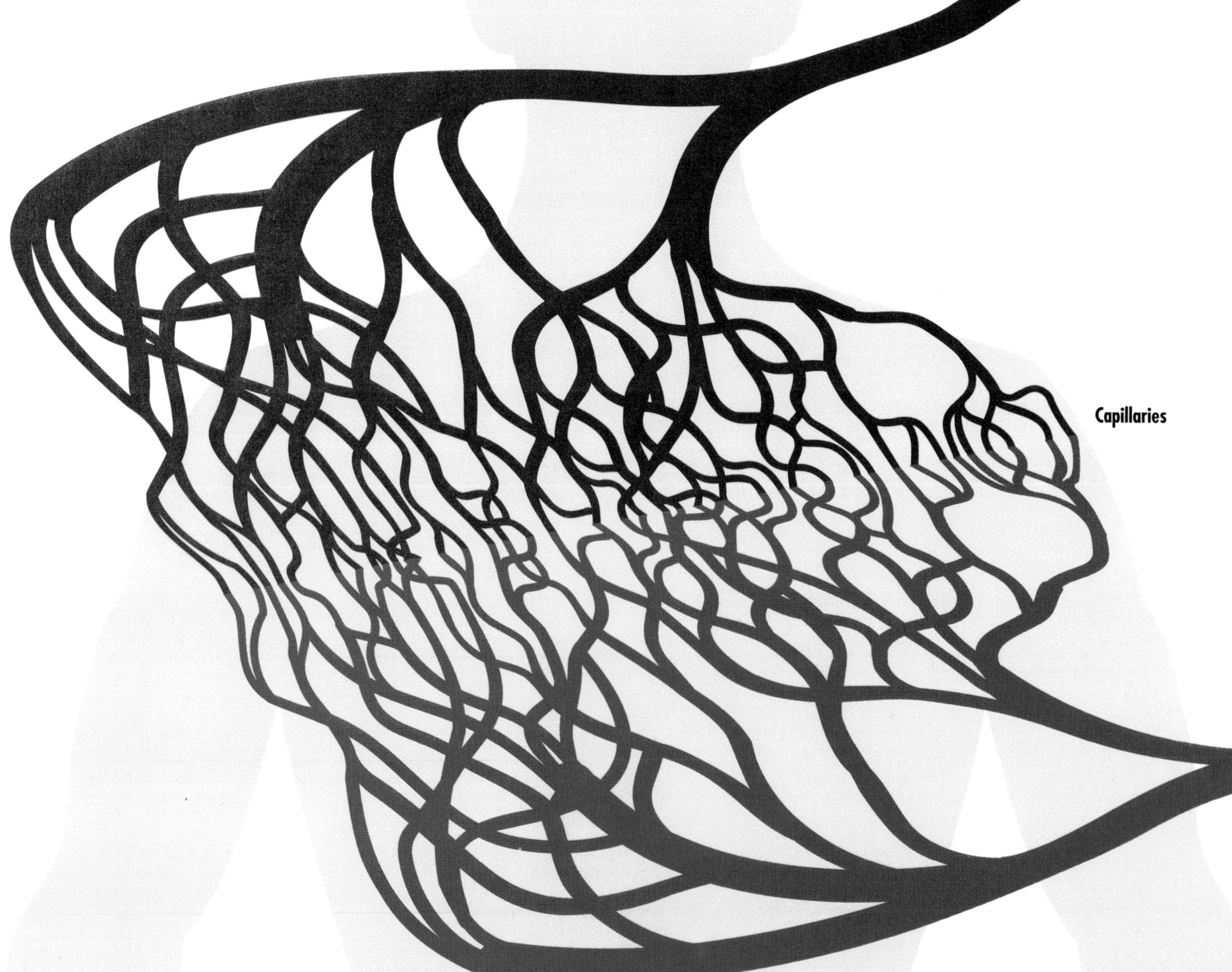

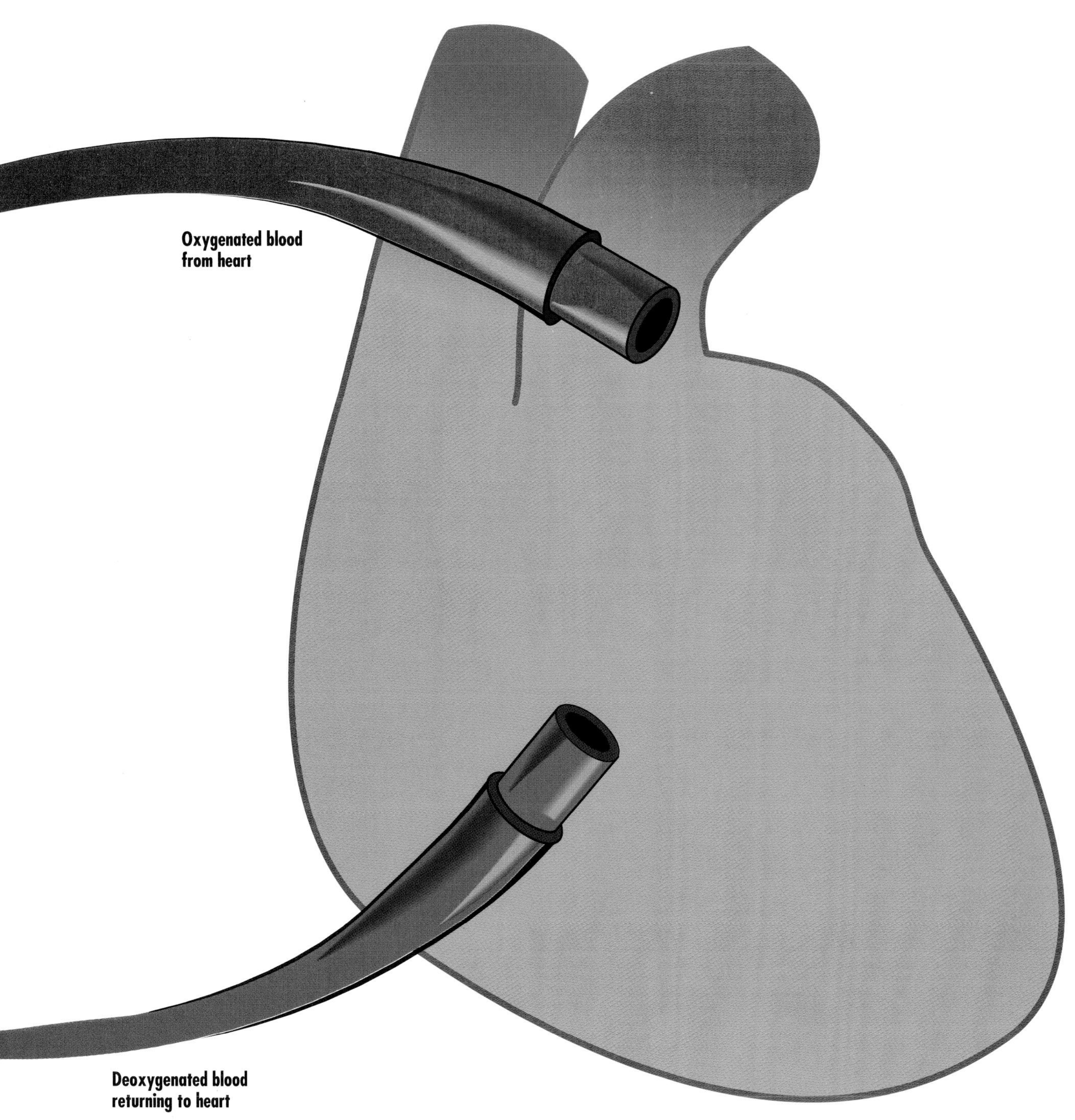
Oxygenated blood
from heart
Deoxygenated blood
returning to heart

# Capillary Circulation

Fluids, oxygen, nutrients, and other substances pass from the capillary blood into the fluid surrounding the cells at the tissue level. Several mechanisms operate to allow this to happen. There are pores and clefts in the capillary wall, and in some instances transfer occurs by bubbles or vesicles crossing the capillary wall. The primary process, however, is diffusion. This is illustrated by the exchange of oxygen, where there is an exchange from the high concentration of oxygen in the capillary blood to the low concentration in the tissues. Simultaneously, the reverse takes place in the lungs, where carbon dioxide diffuses or disperses from the pulmonary capillary system in exchange for oxygen.

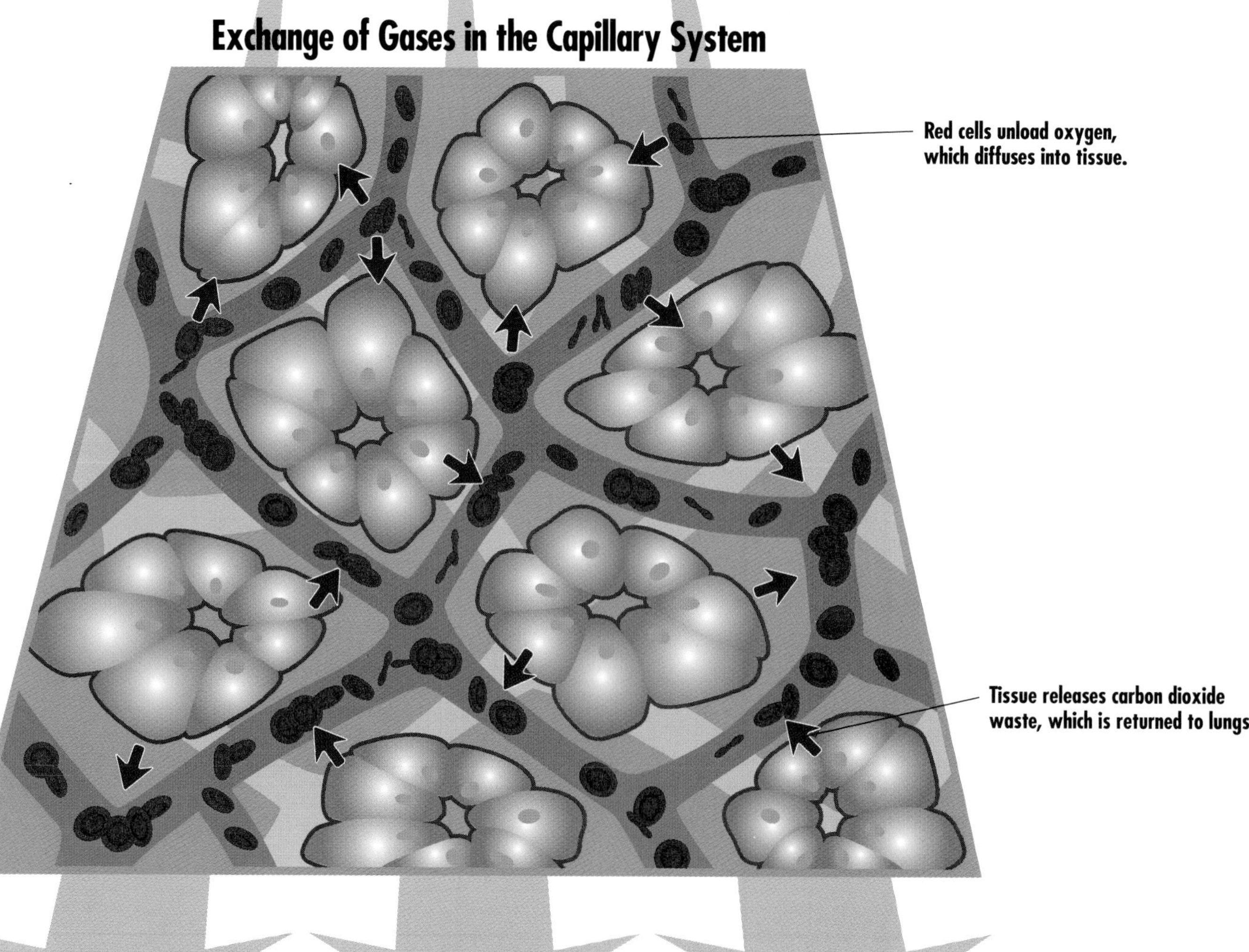

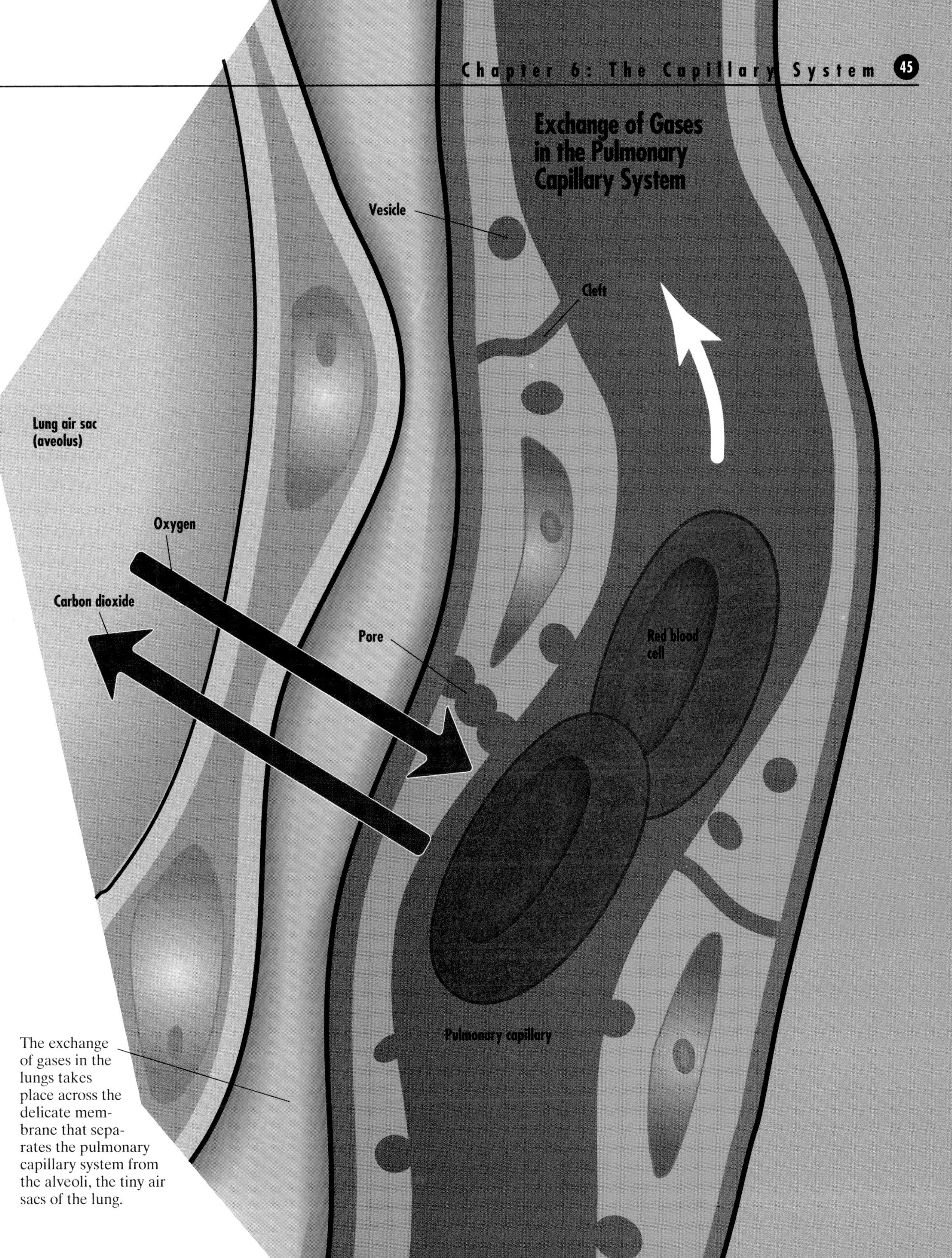


The exchange of gases in the lungs takes place across the delicate membrane that separates the pulmonary capillary system from the alveoli, the tiny air sacs of the lung.

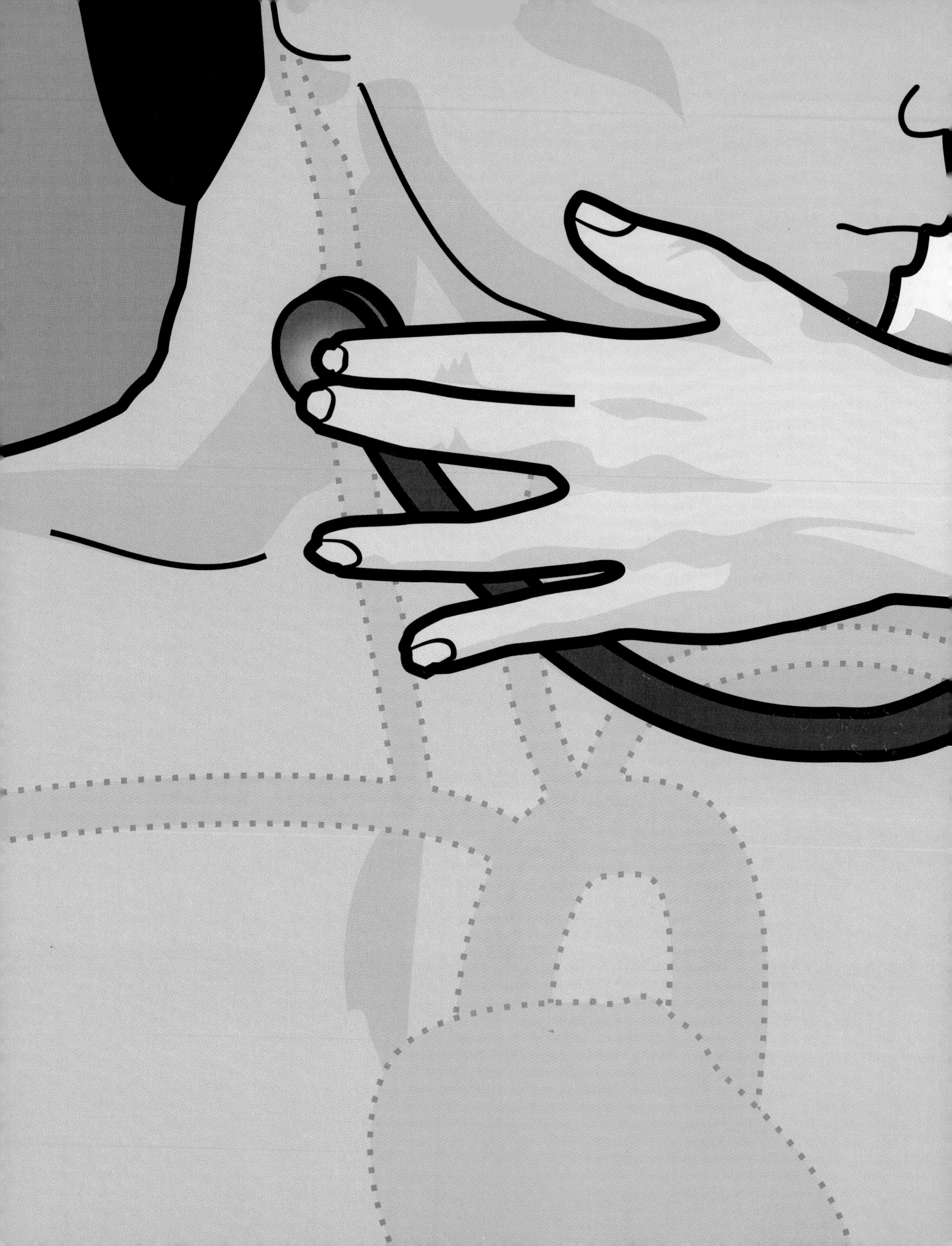

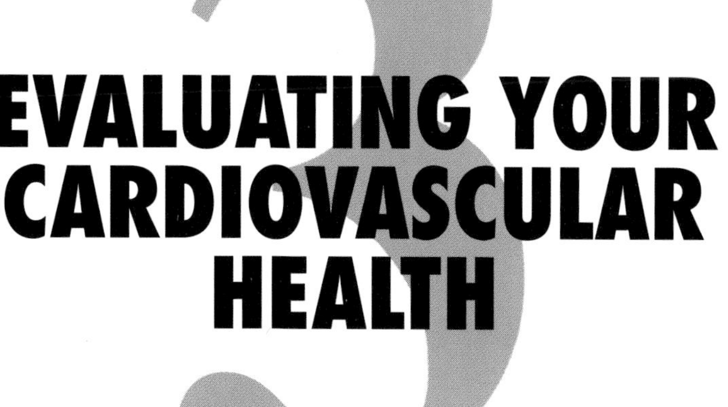

# EVALUATING YOUR CARDIOVASCULAR HEALTH

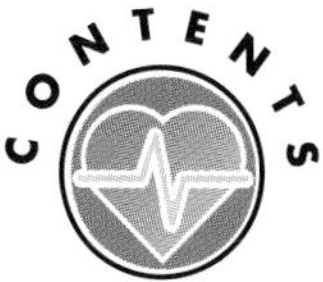




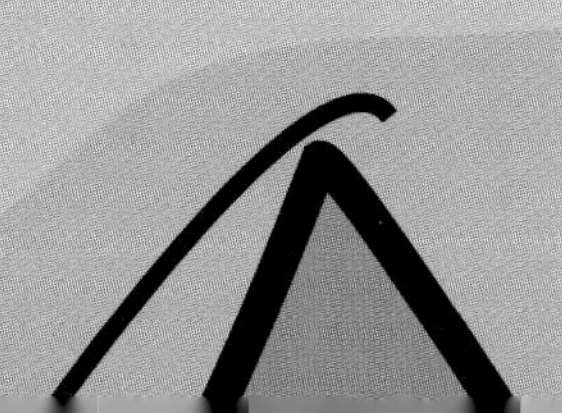

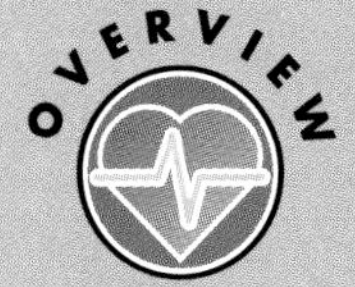

RECENT CHANGES IN the health care delivery system in the United States have resulted in some alterations in the traditional one patient–one physician relationship. An increasing number of individuals use Health Maintenance Organizations (HMOs), multiphysician medical clinics, or hospital emergency departments for their primary medical care needs. Additionally, the many important technologic advancements that have been made in medicine over the last few decades have resulted in a marked increase in specialized medical services. As a result, it is not unusual for a patient to go directly to the specialist involved with his or her disorder. Thus, the cardiac patient may go directly to a cardiac clinic or to a cardiologist without a referral from a primary care or family physician.

However, in spite of the changing nature of the delivery of health care, and no matter who is providing the medical care, the fundamental principles of the medical examination have remained the same over the years. The cornerstones of the initial medical visit are the taking of the medical history and the physical examination. With the information acquired as a result of these two basic components, the physician can almost always make a presumptive diagnosis. The physician then has at his or her disposal a multitude of aids in the form of laboratory tests and special procedures that will establish the diagnosis and enable the physician to prescribe a plan of therapy. This process often requires a team of consultants and technicians as well as special facilities and possibly hospitalization.

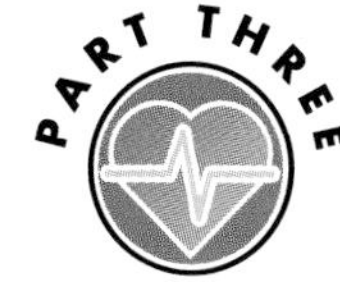


In order for the physician to be able to diagnose a disorder and treat the patient in the most effective way possible, the patient–physician relationship must be one of mutual trust and respect. This requires the utmost cooperation on the part of both parties. For his or her part, the patient must be honest in terms of both information and questions, and also compliant with the physician's advice and recommendations. The physician, in turn, must demonstrate understanding and patience, bearing in mind that the patient may be concerned and even frightened by the threat of serious illness. The patient is always free to obtain a *second opinion,* or more, if dissatisfied with the present relationship or if it is necessary to confirm the diagnosis and plan of treatment because of financial or insurance constraints.

In Chapter 7 we will discuss the medical examination. Chapters 8 and 9 will describe the use of the electrocardiogram and the special procedures that are available to the physician and patient, especially as they relate to the cardiovascular examination.

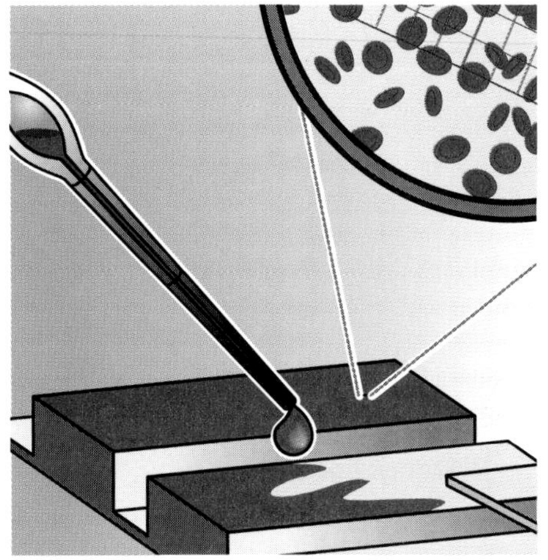

# The Initial Cardiovascular Examination

THE MEDICAL EXAMINATION is vital not only for the information it reveals, but for the establishment of the patient-physician relationship. Through the taking of the patient's medical history and the physical examination, the foundation of mutual trust and respect is laid for building this important relationship. Most physicians have established a standard procedure for the procurement of a patient's medical history. A checklist or interview with a nurse or office personnel will often be used initially to obtain basic personal information such as date and place of birth, occupation, and medications being taken. Remember that aspirin, oral contraceptives, vitamins, and health food supplements are considered medications! The family medical history also may be elicited in this fashion or obtained by the physician. Ages of parents and siblings, living or dead, and causes of death will be included in the family history, as well as history of certain disorders such as diabetes, peptic ulcer, coronary artery disease, and hypertension that may have occured in other family members. Women will be asked about pregnancies, the use of contraceptives, and any obstetric problems or complications.

The history of previous illnesses is an important component of the medical history. In addition to the usual childhood diseases, you may be asked about allergies—especially to medications—and certain specific problems such as rheumatic fever, hepatitis, and procedures such as blood transfusions. You will be asked about current and past smoking habits. In private, the physician may inquire about alcohol intake, sexual orientation, and drug use. The increasing incidence of the Acquired Immune Deficiency Syndrome (AIDS) prompts these questions as well as the history of previous blood transfusions. Answers to all questions are protected by the confidentiality of the medical record.

After obtaining your past and family history, the physician will proceed to the present problem, usually referred to in the medical record as the *chief complaint.* He or she will then obtain a *history of the present illness.* In order to gain as much information as possible about the present illness, the physician will ask many questions and the patient should attempt to answer them as completely and accurately as possible. For example, if the chief complaint is chest pain, the physician will ask about such things as its character (sharp, dull, pressing, etc.), whether it's continuous or intermittent, what brings it on, what relieves it, and if there are associated symptoms such as shortness of breath or a cough. The physician may inquire about symptoms related to other body systems such as indigestion, changes in bowel habits, menstrual disorders, urinary tract difficulties, sleep patterns, and nervousness. All of your responses help guide the physician to a "presumptive" diagnosis.

When your medical history is completed, the physician will give you a physical examination. The extent of the examination will vary, depending on the circumstances. A complete physical examination is essential on your first visit to a physician. This should include an examination of all of your body systems from head to toe, with the possible exception of the female pelvic examination, which is usually left to the expertise of a gynecologist. Examination of the prostate in male patients by rectal examination is an important part of the general physical examination.

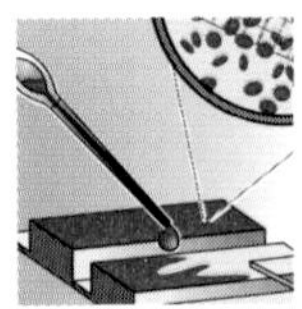

Let's assume that the medical history and general physical examination have led the physician to focus on the cardiovascular system as the source of the patient's problem. Although the heart will command most of the physician's attention, examination of the blood vessels is also included in the cardiovascular examination. Blood pressure will be measured, sometimes both standing and sitting or lying down. Checking the pulses in the feet will provide the physician with a general idea of the status of the larger blood vessels. The physician will listen with the stethoscope over the carotid arteries in the neck for the detection of *bruits*, roughness to the sound of the blood flow due to hardening of the arteries. Close observation of the neck is also useful for evaluating of the veins that reflect heart function. To evaluate the capillaries, the physician may look at the capillaries of the retina and look at the interior of the eyes through an ophthalmoscope.

In examining the heart, the physician will check the chest wall for any abnormal bulges or pulsations. The physician may lay his or her hand on the chest wall to feel for abnormal pulsations. The next part of the examination is an evaluation of the size of the heart by the process of *percussion,* which is tapping the fingers of one hand placed over the heart with the middle finger of the other hand until a change of note is detected. Percussion over the air of the lungs produces a drumlike sound, but at the left border of the heart, the note becomes dull, and the physician can get a rough estimate of the size of the heart. Percussion is also valuable in examining the lungs. The lungs produce the characteristic drumlike noise because of their air content. A change in the percussion note over the lungs suggests something abnormal.

The final portion of the examination of the heart is the procedure of *auscultation,* which is performed with the stethoscope. The stethoscope is simply an audio device that allows the physician to hear body sounds clearly and distinctly. It has an especially valuable place in the examination of the heart, allowing the physician to hear precisely the sounds of the heart as it contracts and relaxes. The physician may ask the patient to assume various positions such as lying on the left side, sitting, or squatting to facilitate auscultation.

The sounds made by the heart have been described fairly accurately as "lubb dup…lubb dup…lubb dup." The first sound, "lubb," is attributable to the contraction of the ventricles and the closing of the mitral and tricuspid valves; the second heart sound, "dup," is related to the closing of the aortic and pulmonic valves. Additional sounds usually, but not always, suggest an abnormality, and may require further analysis by special procedures. Heart *murmurs* are related to the flow of blood through malfunctioning valves that do not open or close properly, either impeding blood flow through a narrowed valve or allowing regurgitation, or backflow, through a loose valve. Auscultation of the heart is also valuable in detecting abnormalities in the rhythm of the heart, or *arrhythmias*, although the physician usually needs help from an electrocardiogram to define the type of arrhythmia.

Auscultation also plays an important role in the examination of the lungs. The sounds of respiration are clear and have a characteristic quality. The stethoscope is valuable in picking up abnormalities in the breath sounds that may have clinical significance and may relate to cardiac disease.

When the history and physical examination are completed, the physician will usually tell the patient the preliminary findings and proceed to fully establish the diagnosis with appropriate laboratory tests and special procedures. These tests contribute to the physician's assessment by supplying information that is not apparent from the physical examination. Usually, the tests serve to reassure the physician that no serious condition exists. Occasionally, results may indicate the presence of a disorder that was not suspected by the physician, and the physician will request other tests or studies to further delineate the problem. In any case, whether results are normal or abnormal, the clinical laboratory will have established baseline values for the individual patient that the physician can always refer to.

Thanks to modern technology, many of these tests, which almost exclusively study a blood specimen, can be performed by automated machines. The most commonly ordered tests are hematology studies that indicate the numbers of different types of blood cells and chemistry studies that indicate the quantities of different compounds in the blood. Over 20 blood tests can be performed on a single specimen of blood. The machine delivers the results on a printout along with normal values and an indication of those values that are outside the normal limits. For example, the physician can obtain information about disorders of the red blood cells such as anemia, as well as disorders of the white blood cells and of the platelets, the small cells that are involved in blood clotting. The results of the blood chemistry studies inform the physician about basic kidney and liver function, the level of blood glucose (sugar), and the levels of electrolytes such as sodium, potassium, chloride, and calcium. If there is an abnormal finding, the physician can now pursue more sophisticated studies to try to pinpoint the cause.

A urinalysis is also done as part of the initial laboratory examination. Depending on the patient's condition, other specimens including sputum and feces may be studied. Testing the stool for blood is an important test that is usually performed when the physician does a rectal examination during the physical examination. With the aid of a specially prepared paper, the presence of hidden blood in the stool can be detected. If positive, the physician will often repeat the test after placing the patient on a meat-free diet for 2 days. If still positive, there is need for further examinations to determine the cause of the bleeding.

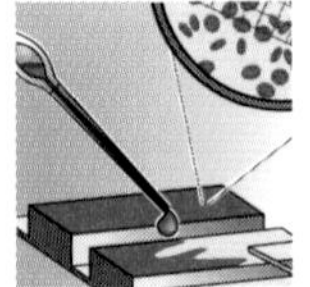

Of the tests related to cardiovascular disease, the level of blood cholesterol is probably the most important study in the laboratory screening procedure. Blood cholesterol is not the villain we often associate with the word. Cholesterol is an essential component of our bodies. It plays an important role in the manufacture of the sex hormones and the hormones excreted by the adrenal glands. Actually, cholesterol is present in every cell of the body, is essential to cell structure, and is manufactured by the cells; this cholesterol is called *endogenous cholesterol.* There is also cholesterol in many of the foods that we eat; this form of cholesterol is called *exogenous cholesterol.* Both types contribute to the cholesterol level of the blood. As we shall see, a high blood level of cholesterol constitutes a serious risk factor for the development of cardiovascular disease and calls for a diagnostic and therapeutic program on the part of the physician. *Hypercholesterolemia,* or high blood levels of cholesterol, tends to run in families, and may be a cause of premature death due to heart attacks. Knowing about cholesterol levels in other family members with heart disease is a good example of the importance of obtaining a family history to assess an individual's risk factors and treatment needs.

For a patient with a high blood cholesterol level, the laboratory can be of further assistance by measuring the different types of cholesterol in the blood. Cholesterol is composed of several components that are structurally distinct from each other and play different roles in the development of *atherosclerosis*. This is the arterial disease that is a forerunner of heart attacks, strokes, and other cardiovascular diseases. There are three main cholesterol components. *High density lipoprotein (HDL)* is "good" cholesterol, which protects against atherosclerosis, and which the physician attempts to increase. *Low density lipoprotein (LDL)* and *very low density lipoprotein (VDL)* are the "bad" cholesterol components, which predispose the patient to atherosclerosis, and which the physician attempts to decrease. The laboratory screening tests will also include a level of the patient's *triglycerides*. These are actual blood fat levels, and high levels may be of significance especially when associated with hypercholesterolemia.

Having done the medical examination and reviewed the results of the general laboratory tests, the physician has formed a preliminary diagnosis and can now proceed with any special tests needed to provide a definitive diagnosis.

# The Cardiovascular Examination

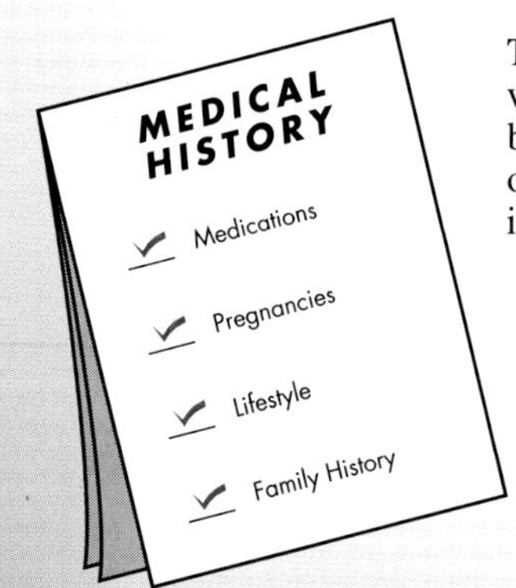


**The Initial Interview** On a patient's first visit to a physician's office, a background of basic information and medical history are obtained. An assistant usually collects this important preliminary information.

**Determining Blood Counts** When a blood count is taken, a small amount of blood is drawn from the sample into a pipette, diluted with a special fluid, and released on a counting chamber. The counting chamber has a grid on it. When examined under a microscope, the number of blood cells on the grid can be easily counted.

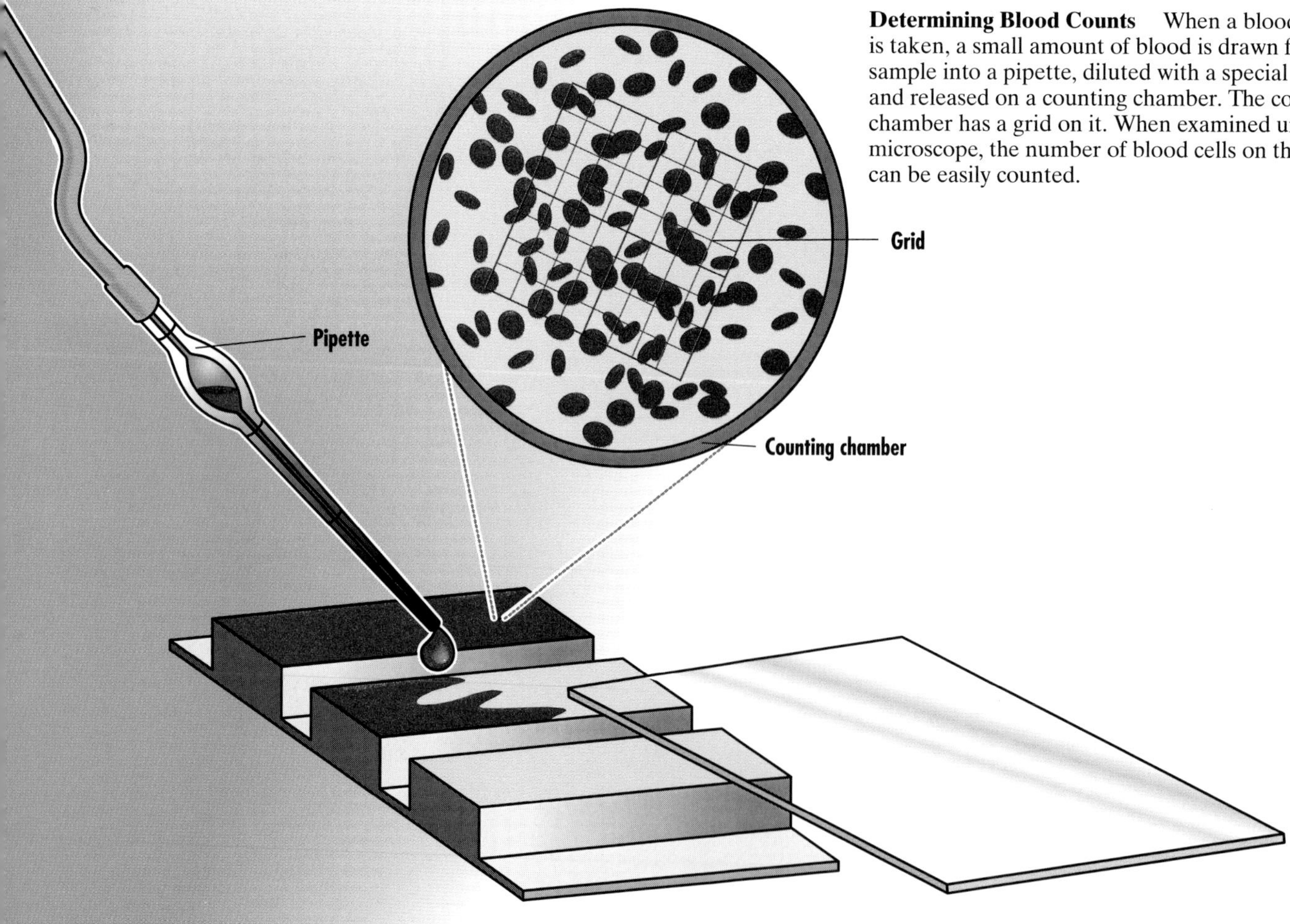

Grid

Pipette

Counting chamber

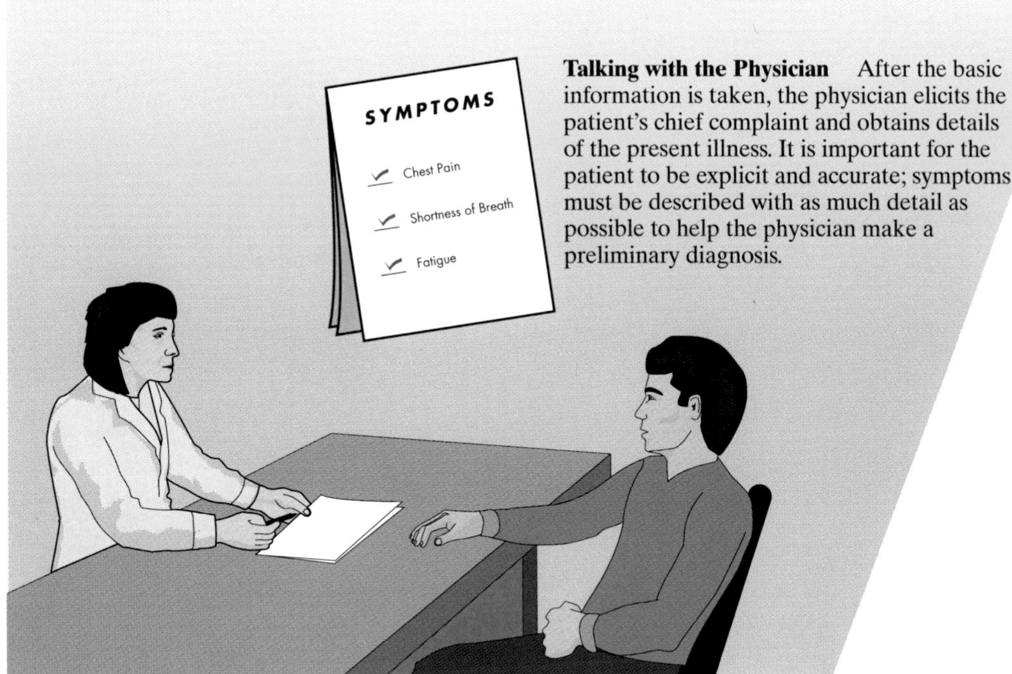


**Talking with the Physician** After the basic information is taken, the physician elicits the patient's chief complaint and obtains details of the present illness. It is important for the patient to be explicit and accurate; symptoms must be described with as much detail as possible to help the physician make a preliminary diagnosis.

**Evaluating the Size of the Heart** The physician places one hand flat on the patient's chest, tapping the middle finger of that hand with the middle finger of the other hand, creating a percussive sound. Over the air-filled lung the sound is drumlike, tympanic and clear. As the hand moves to the border of the heart, the sound becomes flat and dull over the solid tissue of the heart.

**The Physical Examination** Cardiovascular evaluation is a vital part of the physical examination. Part of the evaluation involves the physician using a stethoscope to amplify the heart sounds, enabling detection of abnormalities in the rate and rhythm of the heart beat as well as additional sounds and murmurs. Auscultation of the carotid artery is shown. The insets show how blood flows through an artery with a smooth lining and how it is impeded as it flows past a lining that is rough and jagged because of arteriosclerosis. A hampered flow produces a harsh, grating bruit as the blood passes through.

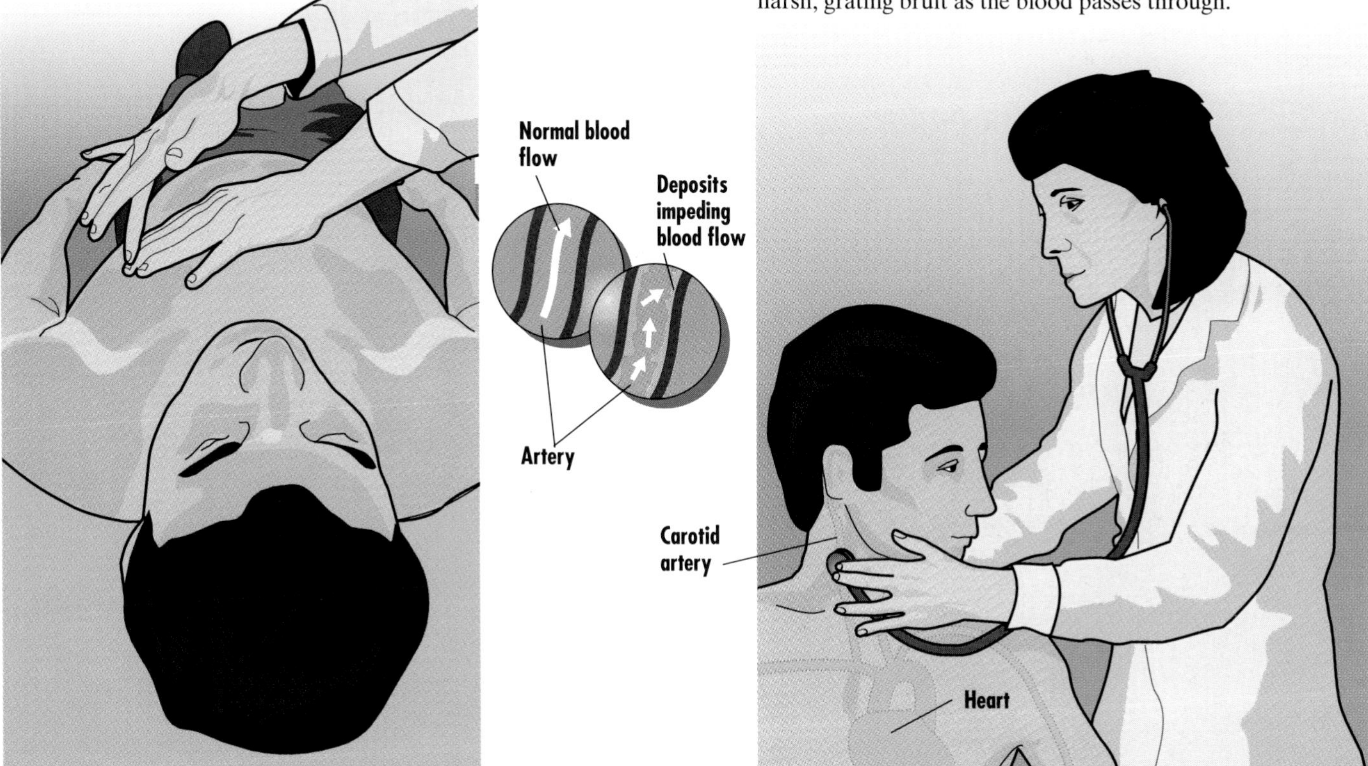

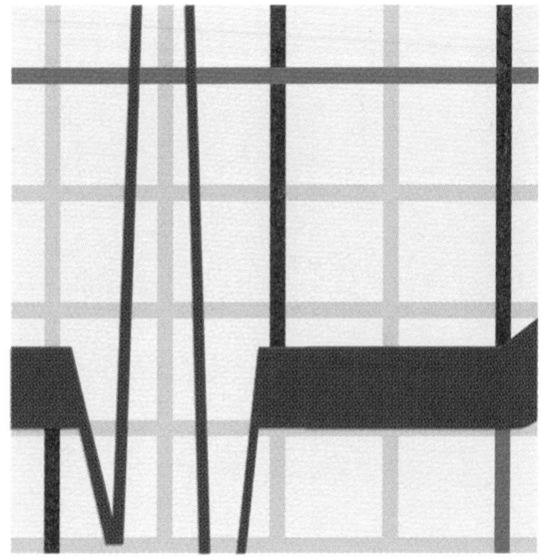

# The Use of the Electrocardiogram

THE ELECTROCARDIOGRAM (ECG) is an indispensable part of medicine. It supplements the physician's information concerning the patient by immediately supplying a visual recording or tracing of the electrical activity of the heart. The electrodes that are placed on the arms, legs, and chest of the patient provide a total of 12 different leads that furnish information on all areas of the heart. Thus, the physician can combine the information gained by the history and physical examination with the ECG results to get a complete cardiovascular analysis.

The ECG provides essential diagnostic information and is especially helpful in monitoring the patient's course and the response to therapy. The ECG is of special value in several particular situations. For example, it is paramount in the diagnosis and treatment of abnormalities of the rate and rhythm of the heart, called *arrhythmias*.

The normal pacemaker of the heart, the sinoatrial (SA) node, produces what is referred to as *normal sinus rhythm*. However, the heart possesses the unique ability to start the electrical impulse that causes the heart to beat at any point along the conduction system. The result is that, under certain circumstances that may or may not be related to underlying heart disease, the normal pacemaker may be replaced by another one at a different site. Blocks or delays may occur in the transmission of the electrical impulse anywhere along the conduction system. Thus, arrhythmias may develop from an abnormal pacemaker in the atria, the atrioventricular (AV) node at the junction of the atria and the ventricles, or in the ventricles themselves. Each one of these sites constitutes an abnormal or *ectopic* pacemaker. An ectopic pacemaker may operate for a single beat or a prolonged series of beats. In some instances, it may become the permanent pacemaker of the heart. The heart rate produced by the ectopic pacemaker may be faster or slower than the normal heart rate and the rhythm produced may be regular or irregular.

Some arrhythmias are more dangerous than others. The simplest and least harmful of the arrhythmias are the extra beats or *extrasystoles* that may arise anywhere along the conduction system. Many individuals have extrasystoles and are unaware of them. *Atrial* extrasystoles have their origin in the atria, and *ventricular* extrasystoles arise in the ventricles. Although single and occasional ventricular extrasystoles do no harm, they are cause for concern if they occur frequently or in prolonged sequences because they result in an inefficient cardiac output that deprives the body of blood and oxygen. For this reason, ventricular arrhythmias require urgent and frequently lifesaving measures to stop them and, if possible, convert them to normal sinus rhythm. Atrial extrasystoles are of little or no clinical significance, but may cause the patient to have palpitation (sensation of rapid or irregular heartbeat). In general, those arrhythmias that do not affect the cardiac output by changes in heart rate or stroke volume are well tolerated by the individual.

It is difficult to state a definite figure concerning which heart rate is so slow that it is considered dangerous. For example, in some well-trained athletes who have developed an increased stroke volume, a rate of 50 beats per minute or less may be adequate. On the other hand, elderly persons or those with heart disease cannot increase stroke volume, and in the presence of a slow heart rate, cardiac output falls. In general, a heart rate of 50 beats per minute or less is cause for concern and requires investigation.

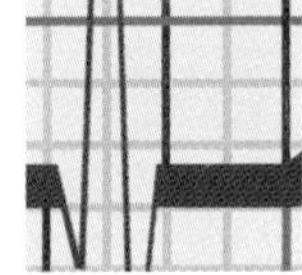

Similarly, the danger from a rapid heart rate is also variable, depending on a person's age and the extent of any cardiac damage. Babies and children routinely have very rapid heart rates of up to 140 beats per minute, which they tolerate quite well. In older people who may have overt or latent heart disease, rapid heart rates may be quite dangerous since they may result in decreased blood supply to the heart muscle and may lower blood pressure, causing neurologic symptoms such as dizziness or fainting. A heart rate of 150 beats or more per minute should be investigated.

One of the major values of the ECG is its assistance in the diagnosis of an acute heart attack or *myocardial infarction.* A myocardial infarction occurs when an area of the heart muscle is deprived of blood because of insufficient coronary blood flow. When this occurs, that portion of the heart muscle dies and the patient is deprived of the function of that portion of the heart. Sudden death may occur if the area of infarction is large and comprises a significant fraction of the total heart muscle. The ECG shows evidence of this condition by the development of abnormal patterns that can be identified by the physician. In many instances, the ECG is the sole diagnostic criterion for discovering a myocardial infarction. The ECG not only aids in making the diagnosis, but also locates the area of the heart where the infarction has occurred.

Taking ECGs at intervals is very helpful in monitoring the course of the patient and evaluating his or her response to treatment. As the patient improves, the ECG shows a gradual series of changes, but usually does not return to normal. The ECG often reveals evidence of a previous myocardial infarction. Aside from its obvious importance in revealing conditions of the heart, the ECG is also valuable as an indicator of certain general body variables such as decreases or increases in the blood levels of potassium, a substance critical to heart muscle function, and certain drugs, especially digitalis, a drug with both important uses in the treatment of heart disease and potential toxicity.

# Understanding Electrocardiograms

The electrocardiogram (ECG) adds valuable information to the diagnostic picture by supplying a visual record, called a tracing, of the heart's electrical activity. These illustrations show ECGs of a normal heartbeat as well as tracings from abnormal heart activity.

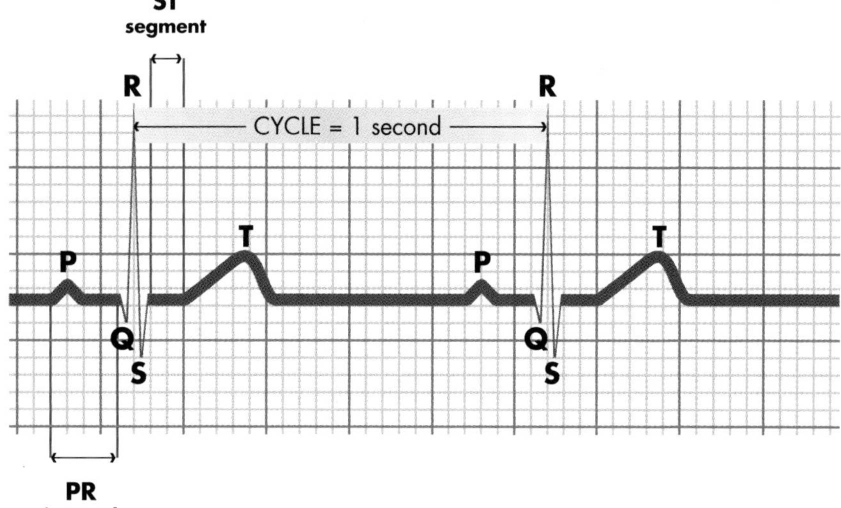


**The ECG of a Normal Heartbeat** The P wave represents the atrial contraction and QRS represents the ventricular contraction. The T wave is produced during the relaxation phase of the ventricle. The time intervals between the ECG components are shown. The time for the entire beat is about 1 second.

**A Rapid Heart Rate** A rapid heart rate of about 150 per minute with a regular rhythm is shown on this graph. The normal appearance of the ventricular complex, the QRS, indicates that the pacemaker is above the level of the ventricles or *supraventricular* in origin, that is, either in the sinoauricular (SA) node or the atrium.

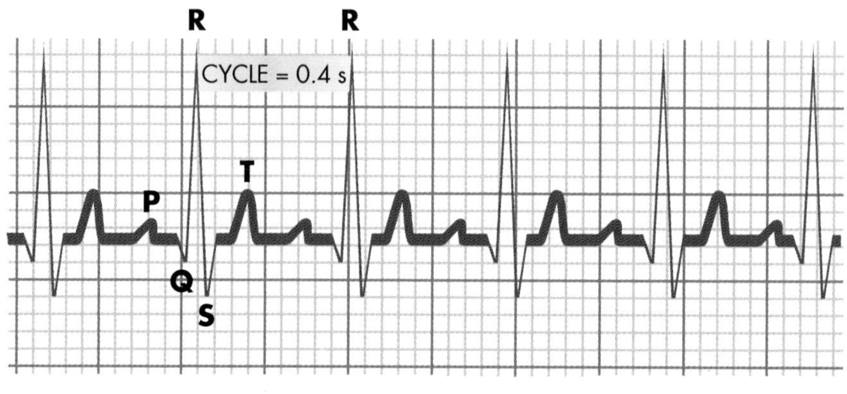

**A Slow Heart Rate** Compare the rapid heart rate ECG with this one of an abnormally slow heart rate of about 50 beats per minute. This slow rate may not provide an adequate cardiac output of blood, especially in elderly patients or in those with heart disease.

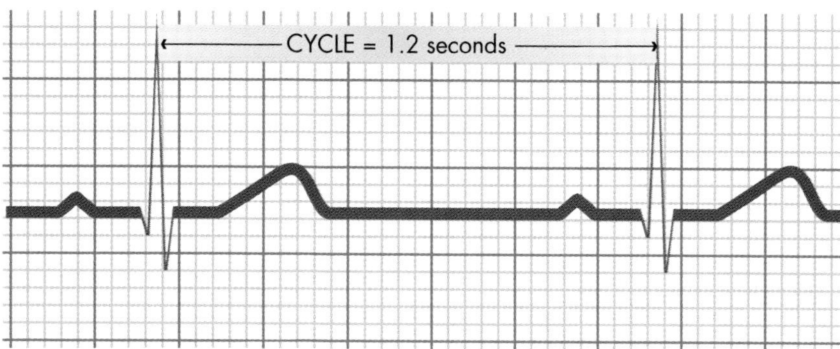


**A Ventricular Extrasystole** The ventricle has become the pacemaker for this one beat causing the premature contraction, a ventricular extrasystole. The QRS complex, representing the ventricular contraction, is widened and abnormal in shape because the impulse did not travel through the normal conduction pathway. Occasional single ventricular extrasystoles occur in many people. They are of no concern unless they occur frequently or in multiples. The asterisk and the arrows represent an abnormal origin of impulse in the ventricle.

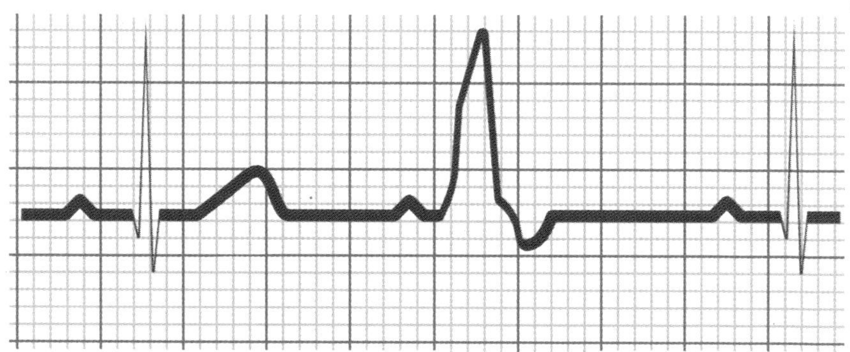

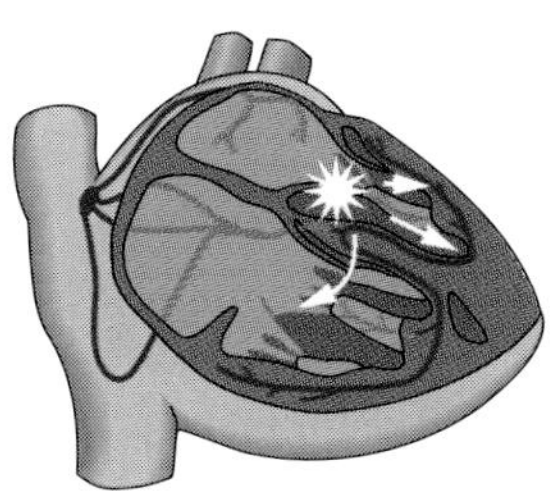

**Ventricular Fibrillation** This ECG shows that the ventricles are twitching with contractions that are feeble and useless in providing an adequate cardiac output. The arrows indicate the abnormal directions taken by the abnormal impulse. This is an extremely dangerous, often fatal, arrhythmia and requires immediate treatment.

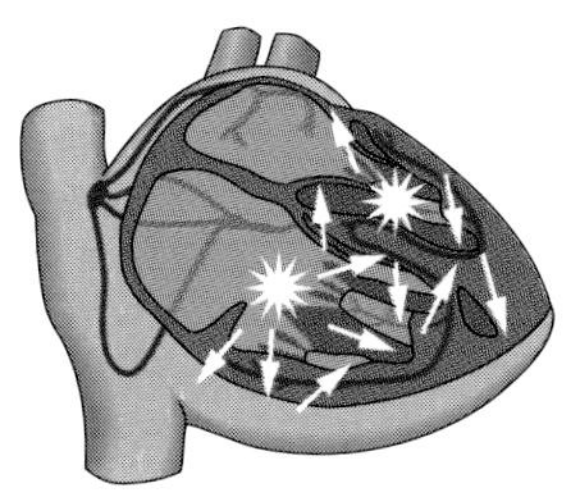

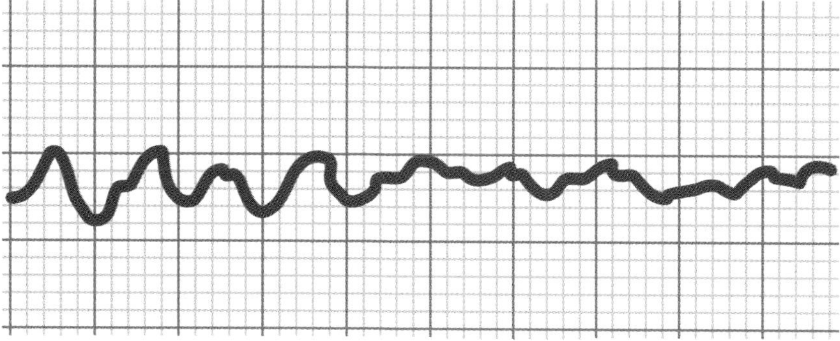

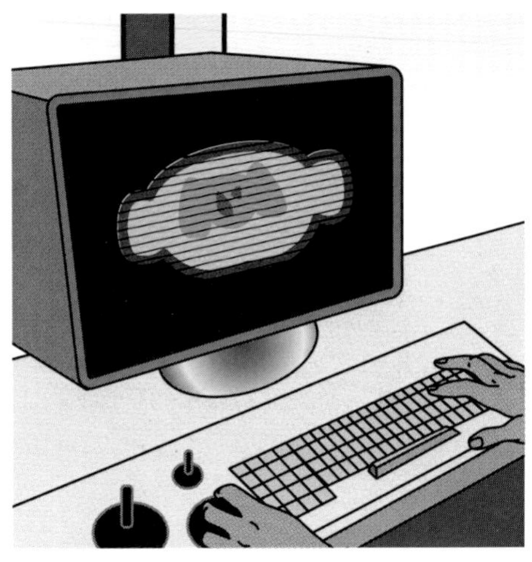

# Special Examinations

IN THIS CHAPTER we will look at several of the more commonly required special examinations. If the physician needs further information after completing the medical history, physical examination, general laboratory tests, and electrocardiogram, he or she has available a number of special studies that will, in most instances, provide the needed information.

A *chest x-ray* is primarily used to determine the status of the lungs. The x-ray is actually the beam used to make the image; the result is a radiograph or roentgenogram, named after Roentgen, the discoverer of x-ray use. Most people, however, use x-ray synonymously with radiograph or roentgenogram. The x-ray also provides valuable information about the size and shape of the heart. Additionally, it helps to define whether shortness of breath, or *dyspnea*, is related to heart disease. Normally, the heart measures less than 50% of the transverse diameter of the chest, that is, the distance from one edge of the chest to the other. Enlargement of the heart indicates the presence of some form of heart disease.

Some physicians prefer to examine the heart directly using the fluoroscope, a component of the x-ray machine that allows direct visualization of the internal structures. This procedure is called *fluoroscopy*. X-ray beams emitted from the x-ray tube pass through the body, producing an image on a fluorescent screen similar to a TV screen. The physician can obtain different views of the heart by using the fluoroscope to examine the patient in various positions. Permanent radiographs or videos can be obtained if desired. Fluoroscopy is painless and takes but a few minutes to accomplish.

Catheterization of the heart, or *cardiac catheterization*, is done by inserting a hollow tube, or catheter, directly into the right or left side of the heart. In difficult diagnostic problems and in evaluating a patient's response to therapy, this study provides important information about pressures within the chambers of the heart and about blood gas concentrations within the heart. This information may be required for a correct diagnosis and often defines therapeutic choices. In right-sided cardiac catheterization, a catheter is inserted into a vein, usually an arm vein, and passed into the right side of the heart. This procedure is particularly useful in diagnosing certain congenital diseases of the heart. In left-sided cardiac catheterization, a catheter is passed into the left side of the heart, usually through a large artery in the groin. Cardiac catheterization often includes the injection of radiopaque dye—dye that is visible on an x-ray—into the cardiac chambers to see the size, shape, and configuration of the heart chambers and valves, as well as their functional status. The test requires up to 3 hours and the patient must be still during this time. A local anesthetic agent is used at the site of the catheterization and the procedure is painless. Sedation may be necessary in children and apprehensive patients.

*Angiocardiography* is a procedure adapted from left-sided cardiac catheterization. It is primarily used to evaluate the condition of the coronary arteries. Under local anesthesia, a catheter is inserted into a large artery, usually in the groin, and then threaded into the aorta and up to the base of the heart. A radiopaque dye is then injected through the catheter, outlining the coronary arteries. A series of x-rays taken in rapid succession provides a video of the filling of the coronary arteries. This procedure enables the physician to study the coronary arteries for areas of narrowing or obstruction. The most important use of angiocardiography is in determining the extent of disease and thus the need for coronary artery surgery such as a bypass or balloon dilation.

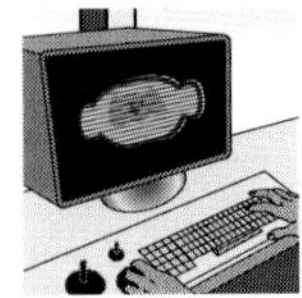

The *stress test* is performed on patients whose symptoms or electrocardiogram suggest coronary artery disease causing insufficient coronary circulation. The test is extremely helpful in identifying those patients who are at risk for worsening symptoms or heart attack due to this insufficiency. The patient is hooked up to an electrocardiograph and steps onto a treadmill. After the treadmill walk is begun, the speed is gradually increased. A physician monitors the patient's pulse and blood pressure as well as the continuous electrocardiogram. The stress test is discontinued after a predetermined time, if the patient complains of chest pain or shortness of breath, or if the electrocardiogram changes show evidence of insufficient coronary artery blood flow.

The stress test is often combined with an injection of a radioactive material, usually thallium, administered intravenously immediately after the completion of the stress test. This procedure is called a *radioactive scan*. Thallium is normally taken up by the heart muscle cells and its uptake is detectable by a scanning device. The patient is scanned immediately after the stress test. Failure of the thallium to reach certain areas of the heart usually means that these areas are not receiving an adequate blood supply. An abnormal thallium scan may indicate the need for angiocardiography.

*Magnetic resonance imaging (MRI)* is a relatively new and important technique that provides the physician with a complete visual image of the heart by making successive "cuts" of the heart without exposure to x-rays. This procedure uses two natural and safe forces—magnetic fields and radio waves. The MRI can penetrate or see through bones to evaluate underlying structures in any level or plane of the body. This is useful in imaging deep structures of the body not otherwise accessible and in creating a three-dimensional view for the interpreter. The MRI is rather noisy but is painless and has no known side effects. The procedure requires 30 to 60 minutes during which the patient is enclosed in a soundproof compartment. A physician and technician monitor the procedure and can communicate with the patient by phone.

*Echocardiography* makes use of ultrasound to render a detailed view of the interior of the heart that defines both structure and performance. It is valuable for assessing the contraction of the heart muscle as well as the functioning of the heart valves. Painless and noninvasive, it is frequently used to diagnose and evaluate congenital heart disease. Echocardiography is actually an adaptation of the sonar devices used to detect submarines and other underwater objects. It explores the heart with high-pitched, or ultrasonic, sound waves that are inaudible to the human ear. These sounds, produced and elicited by a hand-held transducer, can be focused like light to penetrate a wall of the heart and then to send back an echo from the opposite wall. The ultrasound echoes are directed and converted into an image on a video screen and a permanent tape record. The echoes thus create a shadowy cross section of the interior of the heart from any angle.

# Special Examinations

**Right-sided Cardiac Catheterization** A hollow tube, or catheter, is inserted into an arm vein and the catheter is passed into the right side of the heart. Instruments inserted into the catheter enable the physician to determine pressures within the right atrium and ventricle. Blood gases—oxygen and carbon dioxide—can also be measured. A radiopaque dye, one that is visible on a radiograph, may be injected to outline the heart chambers and valves. In catheterization of the left side of the heart, the catheter is inserted into an artery, usually in the groin, and passed up the aorta into the left side of the heart where the same procedures can be performed.

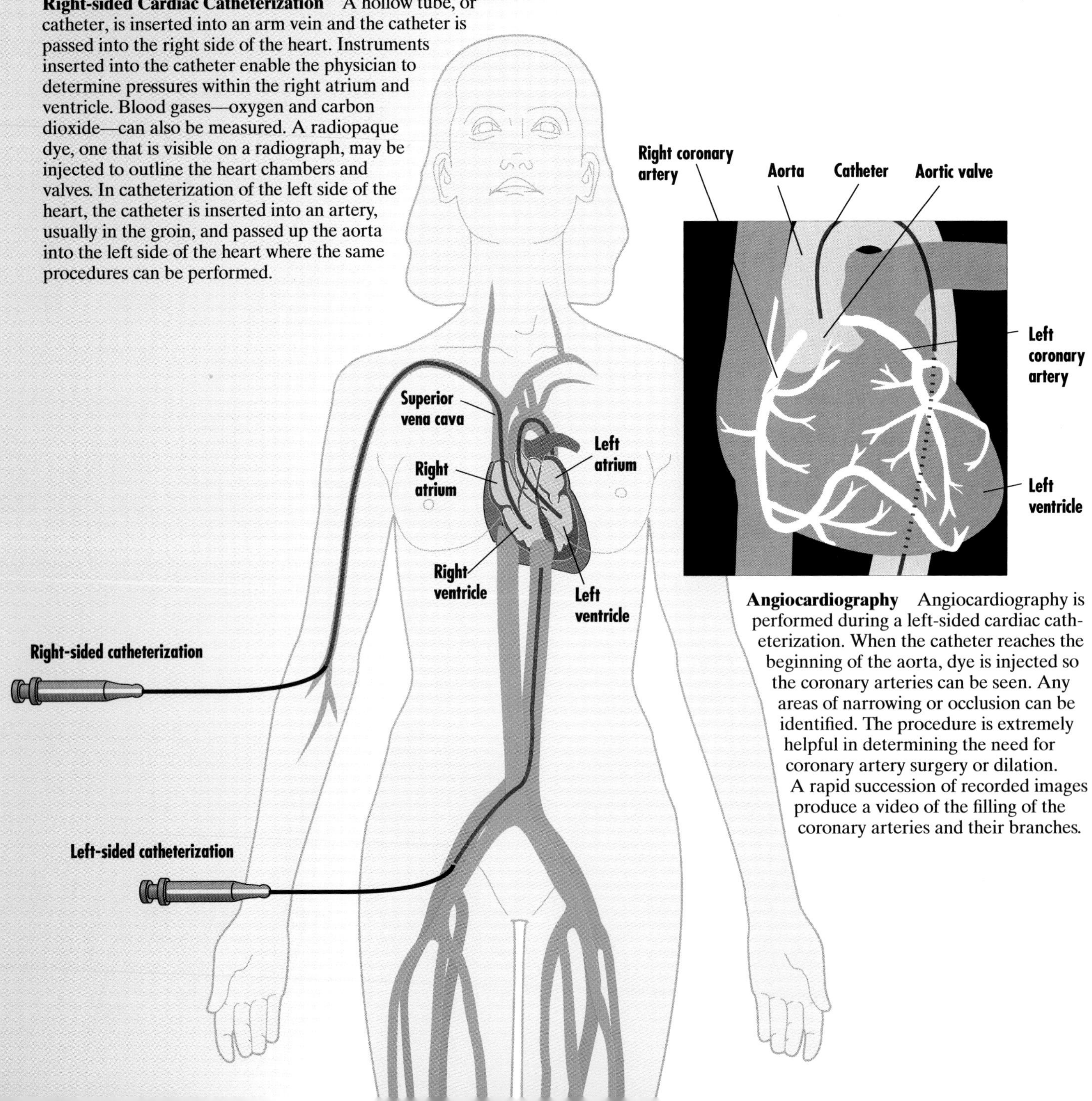


**Angiocardiography** Angiocardiography is performed during a left-sided cardiac catheterization. When the catheter reaches the beginning of the aorta, dye is injected so the coronary arteries can be seen. Any areas of narrowing or occlusion can be identified. The procedure is extremely helpful in determining the need for coronary artery surgery or dilation. A rapid succession of recorded images produce a video of the filling of the coronary arteries and their branches.

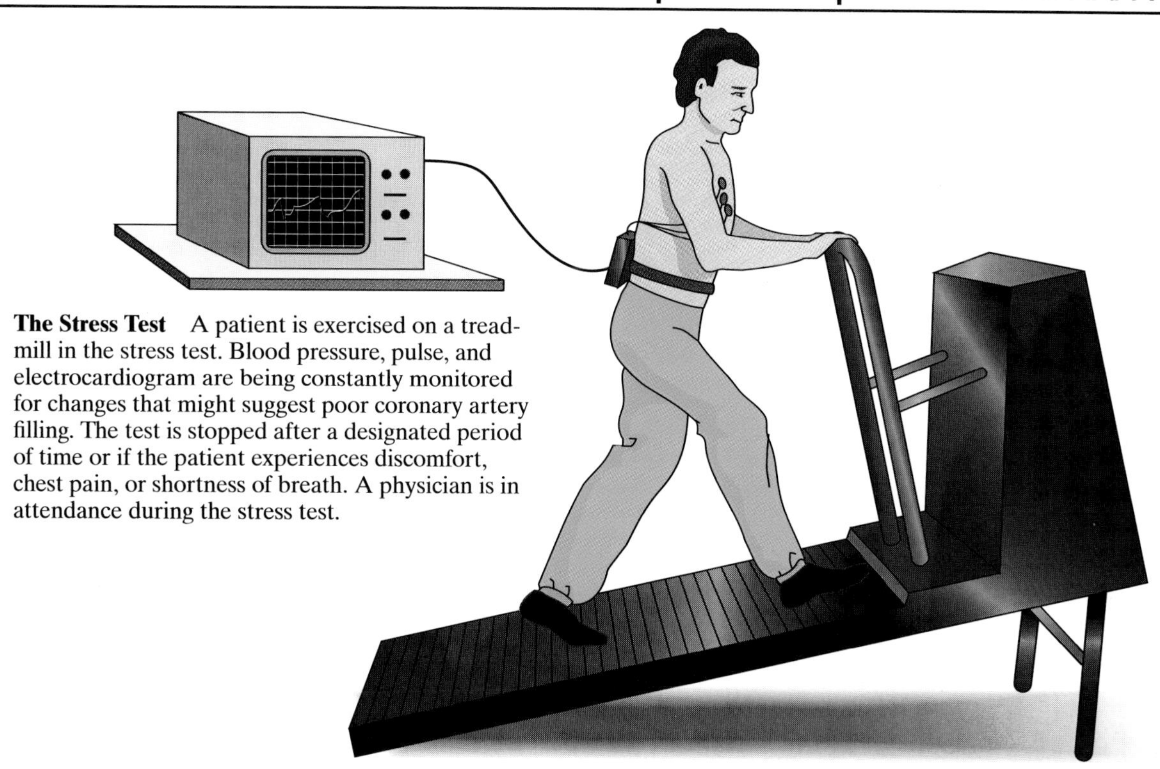

**The Stress Test** A patient is exercised on a treadmill in the stress test. Blood pressure, pulse, and electrocardiogram are being constantly monitored for changes that might suggest poor coronary artery filling. The test is stopped after a designated period of time or if the patient experiences discomfort, chest pain, or shortness of breath. A physician is in attendance during the stress test.

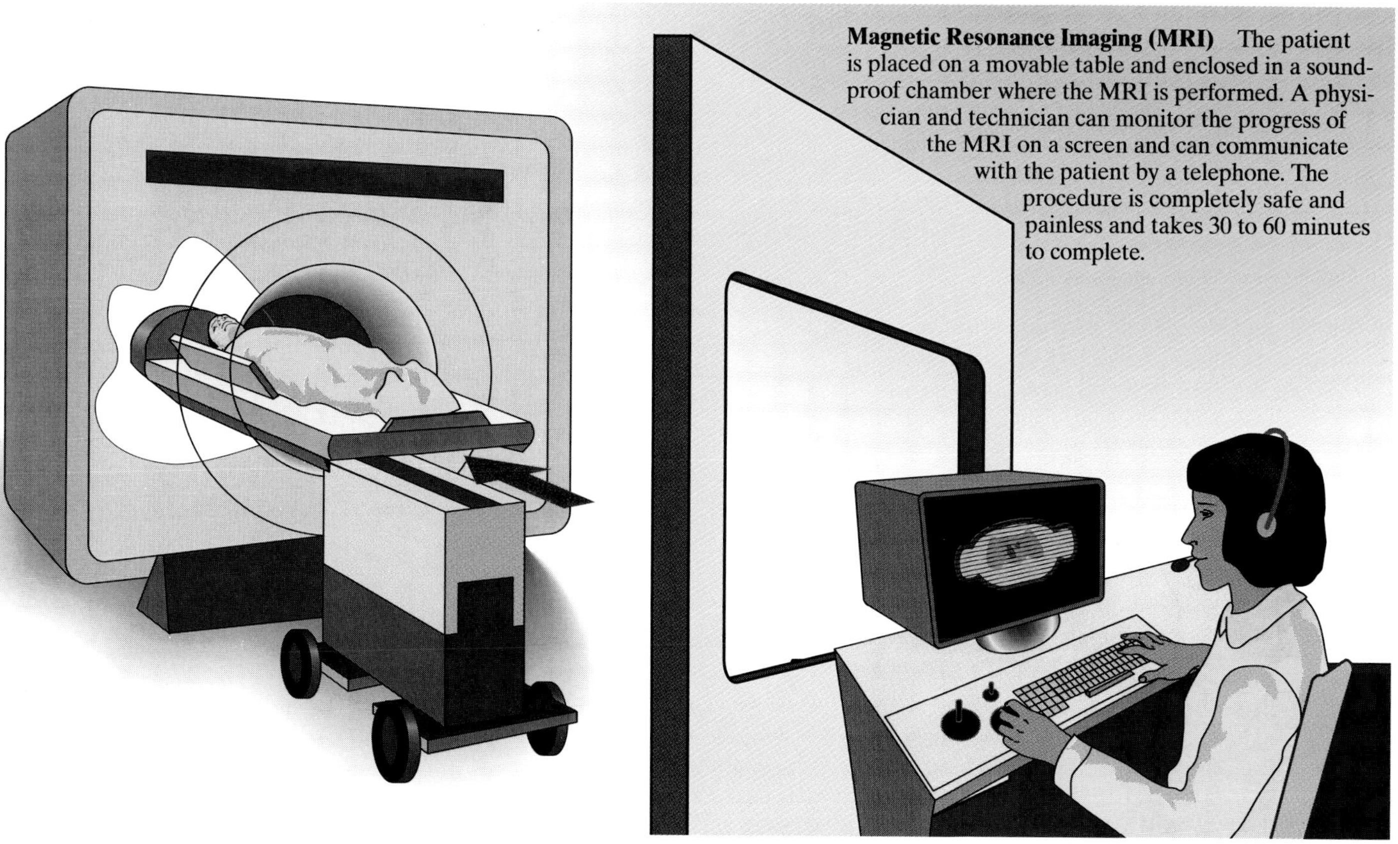

**Magnetic Resonance Imaging (MRI)** The patient is placed on a movable table and enclosed in a soundproof chamber where the MRI is performed. A physician and technician can monitor the progress of the MRI on a screen and can communicate with the patient by a telephone. The procedure is completely safe and painless and takes 30 to 60 minutes to complete.

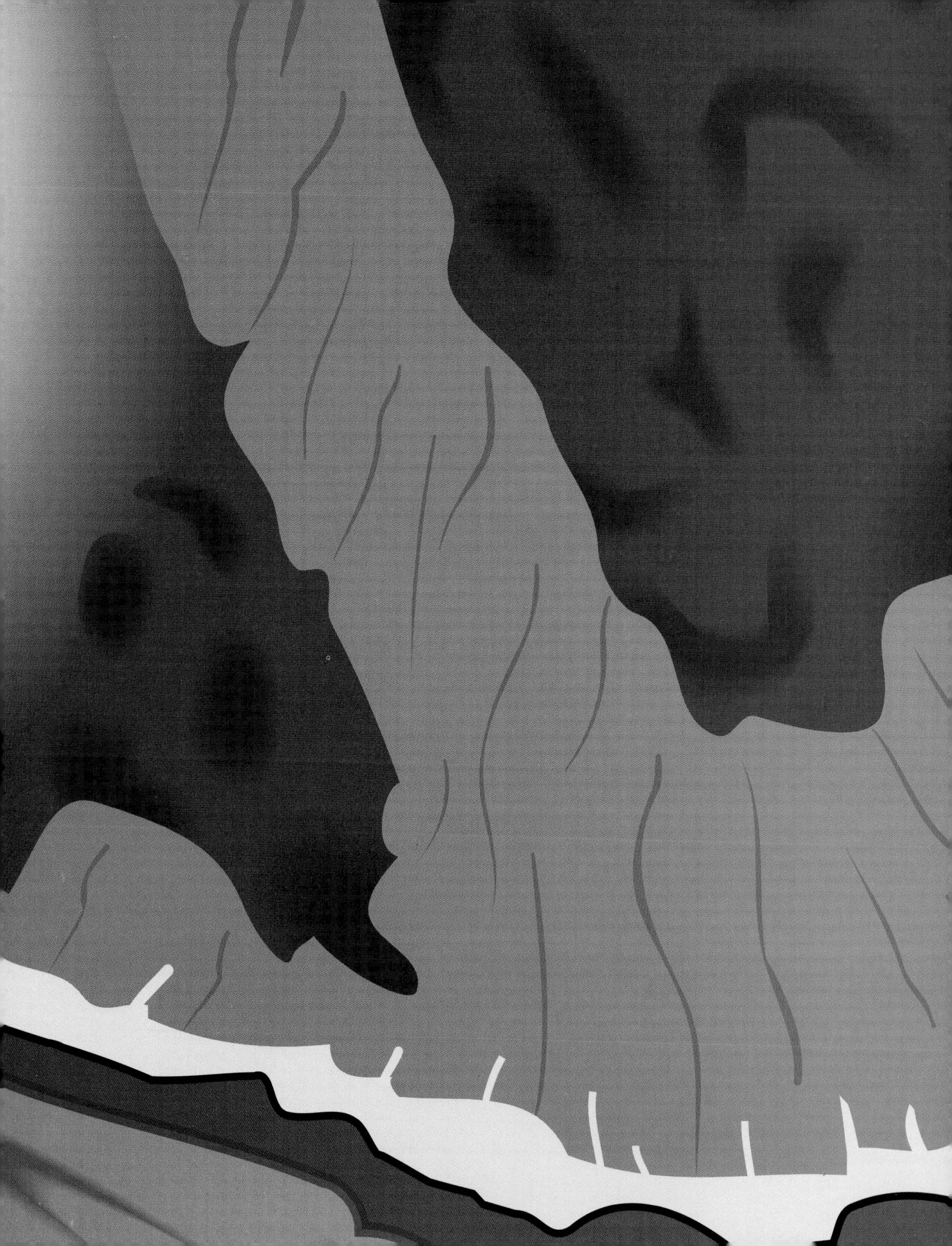

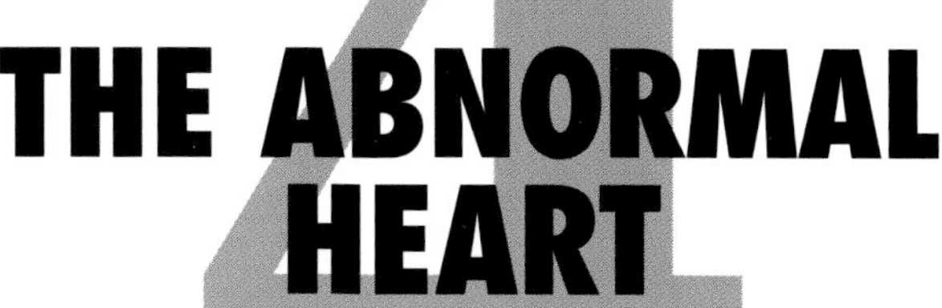

# THE ABNORMAL HEART

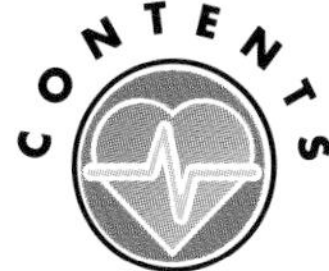

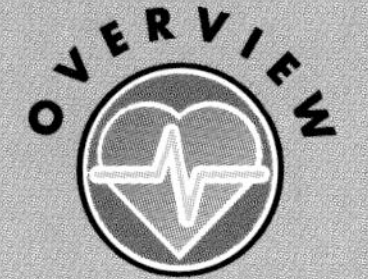
OVERVIEW

IN PREVIOUS PARTS of this book we have concentrated on the anatomy and physiology of the normal heart and the methods and means by which the physician can evaluate the status of the heart. We also discussed how the physician can make an accurate diagnosis of cardiovascular disease. Emphasis has been placed on the importance of the medical history and the physician's general and cardiovascular physical examinations. The importance of the electrocardiogram has been discussed, and we have briefly described some of the special studies that are available to the physician for the evaluation of the cardiovascular system.

We now turn our attention to the abnormal heart, and in subsequent chapters we will review the main categories of heart disease, which include congenital heart disease, congestive heart failure, coronary heart disease, valvular heart disease, and infections of the heart. We will discuss the abnormal anatomy and physiology of these disorders and will describe the characteristic abnormal findings in the medical history, physical examination, electrocardiogram, and other studies that help the physician establish the diagnosis and plan therapy.

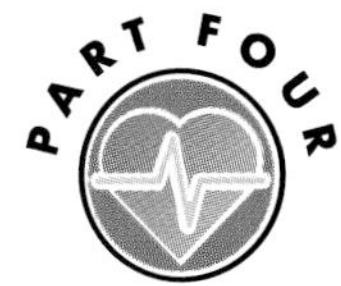

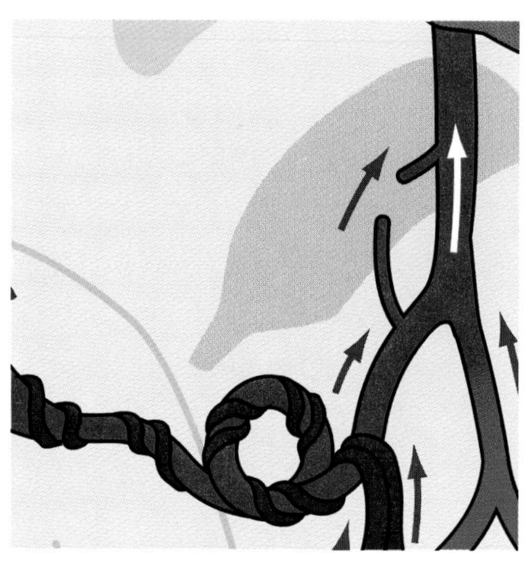

# Congenital Heart Disease

THE DEVELOPMENT OF the cardiovascular system during fetal life is extremely complex. It is not surprising, therefore, that a serious form of congenital heart disease occurs about once in every 125 births (0.8%). Based on this incidence, about 32,000 babies are born each year with some form of congenital heart disease. The word *congenital* indicates that the condition, regardless of the cause, is present at birth. It is distinguished from the term *hereditary*, which indicates that a condition is genetic, that is, transmitted through parental genes. Hereditary forms of heart disease are extremely rare. Thanks to modern technologic advances that make possible prompt diagnosis and improved surgical procedures, definitive methods of medical and surgical treatment for most congenital cardiovascular conditions are now available.

Some congenital disorders result from persistence of the fetal cardiovascular system. We have seen that after birth all venous blood passes from the right heart through the lungs for oxygenation and returns to the left heart for systemic circulation. During fetal life, however, there is no gas exchange occurring in the lungs because the fetus is not exposed to the environment and is not breathing in the true sense of the word. Oxygenated blood is supplied to the fetus by the maternal circulation.

Two structures operating during fetal life allow the circulation to bypass the lungs. They result in a direct flow of maternal oxygenated blood to the arterial system, the so-called right-to-left shunts. One of these is the *foramen ovale*, an opening between the right atrium and the left atrium; the other is the *ductus arteriosus*, a blood vessel connecting the pulmonary artery and the aorta. Both of these structures allow maternal oxygenated blood to bypass the lungs and enter the arterial system directly. Both structures normally close after birth when blood flows through the lungs after the baby begins breathing.

If the ductus arteriosus fails to close, a condition called *patent ductus arteriosus*, the normal higher pressure that soon develops in the left side of the heart and the aorta reverses blood flow in the ductus, and blood flows from the aorta into the pulmonary artery. In other words, the shunt changes its direction from a right-to-left to left-to-right shunt. This, in turn, causes an excessive amount of blood flow to the lungs and then back to the left heart. The heart is eventually unable to tolerate this increased load and there is failure of the left ventricle's pumping action, a condition known as *congestive heart failure*. The diagnosis of patent ductus arteriosus is suggested by the presence of a characteristic murmur over the area of the ductus. Confirmation of the diagnosis is made by echocardiogram or cardiac catheterization. Surgical correction of a patent ductus arteriosus is done by cutting the vessel and sealing off both ends.

The most common congenital cardiac abnormality is a defect in the wall or septum that separates the left and right ventricles. This is called a *ventricular septal defect* (*VSD*) and also results in a shunt of blood from the high-pressure left ventricle to the low-pressure right ventricle. The consequences are similar to those of patent ductus arteriosus—an increase in the volume of pulmonary blood flow followed by overload of the left ventricle with resultant pump failure. The diagnosis is suggested by the presence of a harsh murmur that is caused by the flow of blood through the defect. Confirmation of the diagnosis is made by echocardiogram or cardiac catheterization. Surgery can be used to successfully close the shunt.

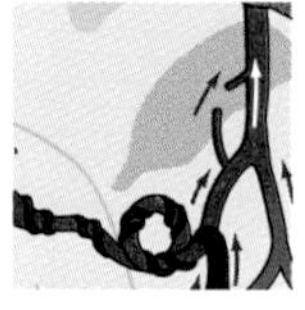

Some congenital heart diseases result in inadequate pulmonary blood flow or the entrance of poorly oxygenated blood into the arterial circulation. The main manifestation of this is *cyanosis*, a bluish discoloration of the skin and membranes due to high concentrations of poorly oxygenated blood. The body attempts to compensate for this condition by producing an excessive amount of red blood cells, a condition referred to as *polycythemia*. Polycythemia, in turn, leads to excessive blood coagulation, a situation that may result in damage to various organs, especially the brain.

Most congenital heart diseases characterized by cyanosis are complex disorders in which the component responsible for the cyanosis is an obstruction to the flow of blood to the lungs leading to decreased blood oxygenation. Depending on the complexity of the individual situation, some form of corrective surgery may be possible.

Structural abnormalities that allow passage of venous blood into the arterial circulation may also cause cyanosis. This occurs if the foramen ovale remains patent, or open, or there is another defect in the septum between the two atria. A large opening between the two atria allows shunting of deoxygenated blood to such a degree that cyanosis develops. The diagnosis is established by echocardiogram or possibly cardiac catheterization and is correctable by surgery.

Congenital heart disease may involve a variety of defects involving any of the heart valves, either alone or in conjunction with other defects. The valve abnormalities are usually in the form of obstructions to blood flow through the valve, called *valve stenosis* or *atresia*. Stenosis is narrowing; atresia is absence or closure. Any valve or combination of valves may be involved. The clinical findings and the results of studies will vary, depending on which valve or valves are involved and whether they are combined with other defects. Most valvular lesions are correctable by surgery.

Many serious congenital heart diseases involve abnormalities in the heart chambers or in the large blood vessels leading to and arising from the heart. Some of these defects are not amenable to surgery and are incompatible with life. However, in this chapter we have concentrated on the most common abnormalities and those with a good prognosis.

There are variations in the degree of severity of congenital defects, as a result of which each patient poses a different problem. In some instances, the seriousness of the situation calls for immediate surgery. On the other hand, some defects are compatible with a normal life and may be diagnosed as a result of another disorder. For example, a small ventricular septal defect that is causing no serious cardiovascular problem can be left alone indefinitely. Between these two extremes are a number of patients who can be safely observed and surgery can be postponed until the patient is older or until the situation warrants it.

# Congenital Heart Disease

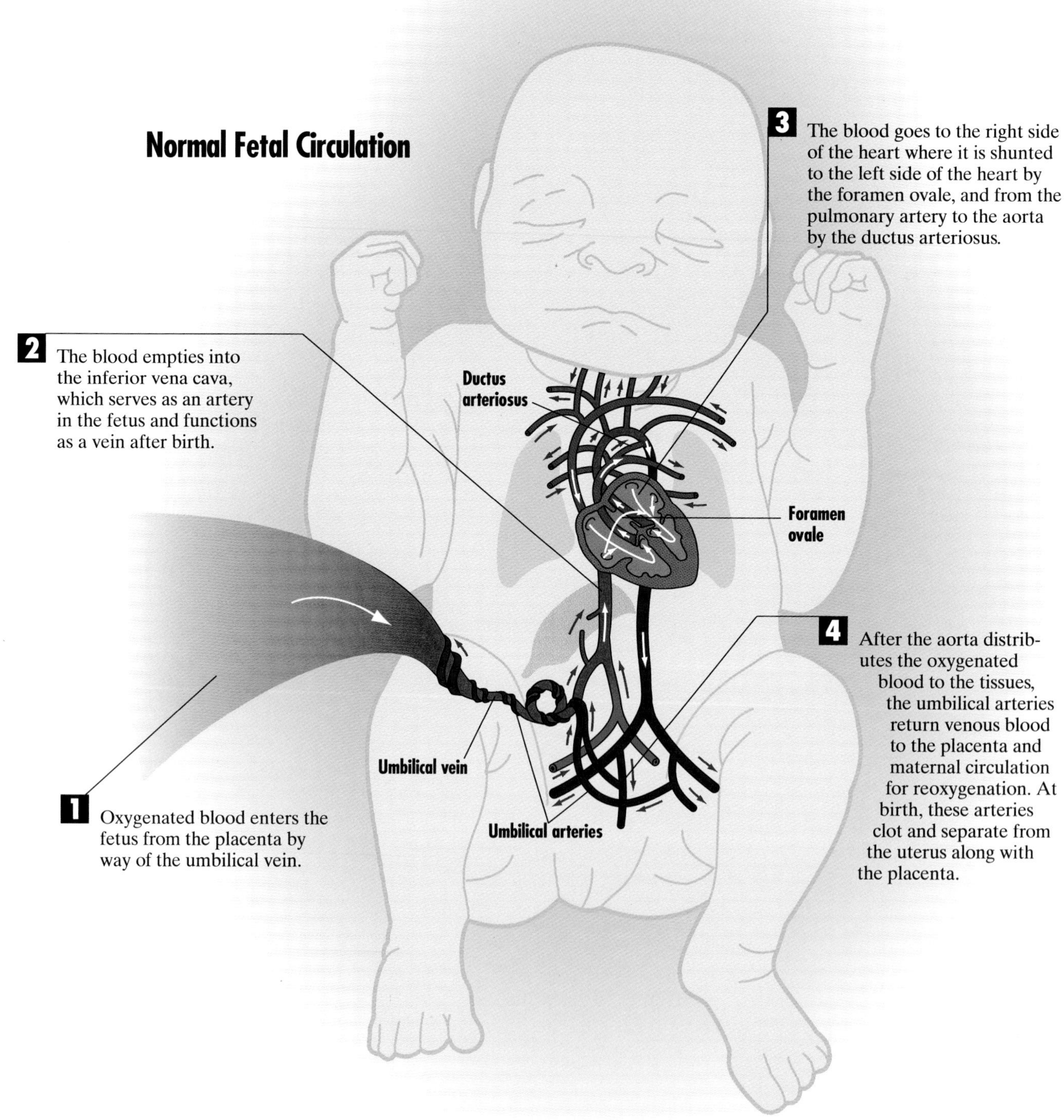

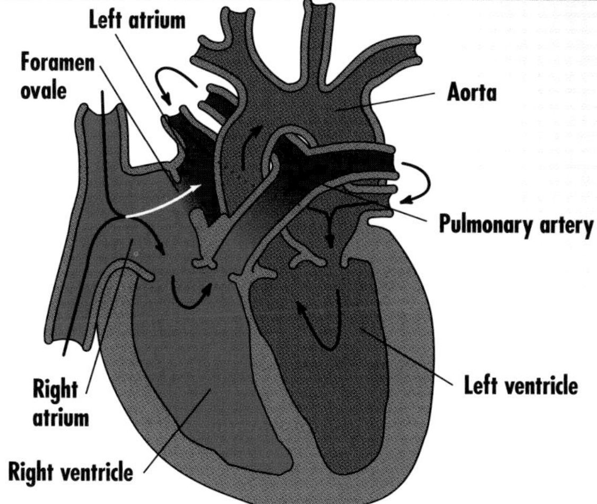


**Patent Foramen Ovale** When the connection between the right and left atria that functions during fetal life fails to close after birth and continues to function, a patent—or open—foramen ovale results. Venous blood flows from the right atrium through the patent foramen ovale into the left atrium and the arterial system. Cyanosis, a bluish discoloration of the skin and membranes due to the high level of poorly oxygenated blood, is the visible result.

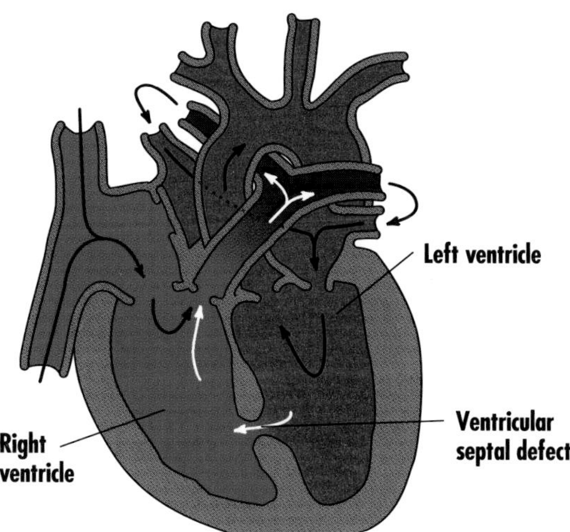


**Ventricular Septal Defect** The septum or wall between the two ventricles sometimes fails to develop fully and a connection between the two ventricles results. The high pressure in the left ventricle forces blood through the defect, causing an increase in the circulation to the lungs. As in the case of patent ductus arteriosus, a large defect eventually places a serious burden on the left ventricle, with resultant pump failure.

**Patent Ductus Arteriosus** During fetal life when the lungs are not functioning to supply oxygen, maternal blood is shunted through the ductus arteriosus into the arterial circulation. If the ductus fails to close after birth, the high pressure that develops in the left side of the heart and aorta causes a shunt of blood from the the aorta to the pulmonary circulation. This overloads the pulmonary circulation and results in an increase of blood returning to the left side of the heart. Eventually, the left ventricle becomes unable to handle this excessive load and there is pump failure. This condition is known as congestive heart failure.

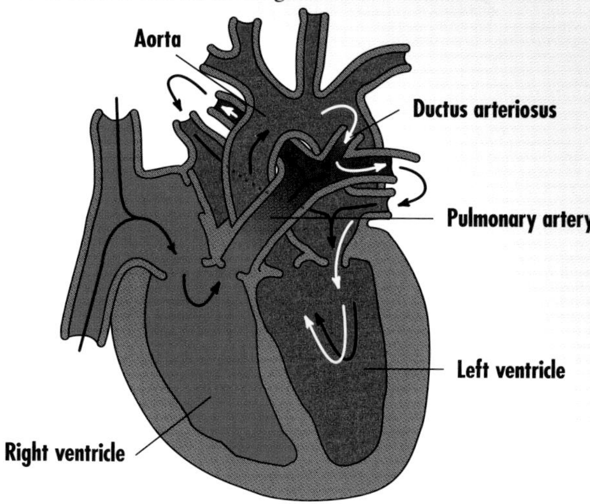


**Congenital Abnormalities of the Aortic Valve** Two types of congenital defects of the aortic valve are illustrated. The bicuspid valve has only two instead of the normal three cusps. A valve with congenital aortic stenosis has cusps that are partially fused, which impedes blood flow through the valve.

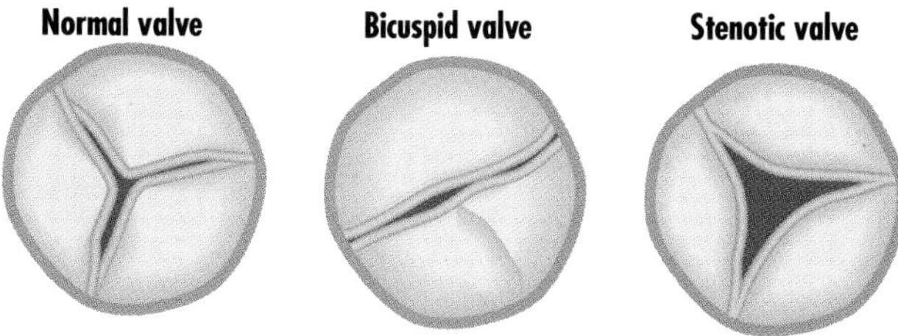

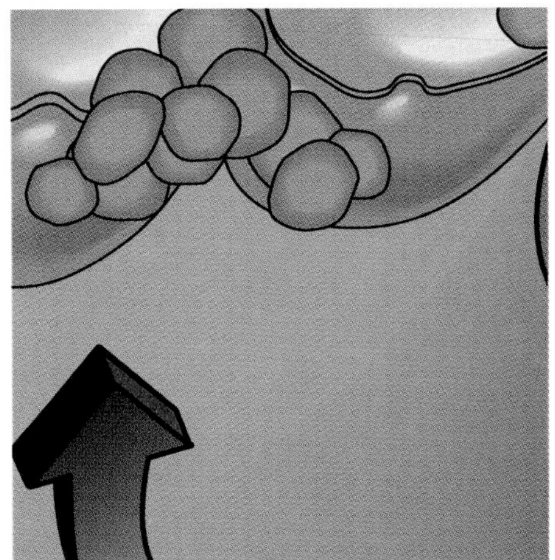

# Congestive Heart Failure

CONGESTIVE HEART FAILURE occurs as a consequence of any cardiovascular disorder that makes the heart unable to perform adequately as a pump and supply body tissues with oxygenated blood and other nutrients.

An important distinction must be made between *acute heart failure* and *congestive heart failure.* Acute heart failure is a sudden, catastrophic condition caused by any cardiac or noncardiac event that arrests effective heart action. It most frequently occurs as a consequence of an acute heart attack, called *acute myocardial infarction,* and a serious cardiac arrhythmia such as ventricular fibrillation. Some examples of noncardiac events that precipitate acute heart failure include massive hemorrhage, severe brain trauma, and electrocution. Acute heart failure requires immediate emergency treatment, but is often fatal even when appropriate therapy is available.

By contrast, congestive heart failure, which we will discuss in this chapter, may occur acutely but more often develops gradually over weeks, months, or even years. A person may live years with congestive heart failure as a chronic condition, managed with medications and regular follow-up. We will discuss several basic mechanisms that can lead to congestive heart failure.

When the cardiac muscle, or myocardium, is diseased, its contractility is impaired and the cardiac output is decreased. Coronary artery disease is the most common cause of myocardial disease. Hardening of the coronary arteries, or *arteriosclerotic heart disease*, reduces blood supply to the myocardium, leading to structural damage and impaired contractility. Infections of the myocardium, *myocarditis,* are also responsible for myocardial failure.

Any process that increases the resistance against which the heart has to pump will strain the myocardium and may result in congestive heart failure. Hypertension, or high blood pressure, is a common example of this mechanism. The left ventricle must perform increased work to overcome the increased resistance due to high arterial pressure. Obstruction of the aortic valve is called *aortic stenosis* and forces the heart to work against increased resistance. Severe lung disease such as emphysema may increase the resistance to right ventricular output and eventually lead to right ventricular failure, a condition referred to as *cor pulmonale.*

Some abnormal conditions increase the volume of blood returning to the ventricles. Examples are congenital heart disease such as patent ductus arteriosus and interventricular septal defect. Heart valve abnormalities that allow backflow or regurgitation of blood into the ventricles also overload these chambers. An important example of this is aortic valve regurgitation, which occurs with defective closure of the aortic valve during diastole. This allows blood to regurgitate from the aorta back into the left ventricle, thus increasing the volume of blood to be ejected and the force required to eject it.

There are some conditions such as infections, anemia, and an overactive thyroid that require an increase in cardiac output. Although any one of these conditions alone rarely causes congestive heart failure, it may contribute to its development given underlying cardiac disease.

The heart has mechanisms to compensate functionally for the underlying cardiovascular disorder stressing it. The myocardium is capable of increasing its muscle mass, thereby increasing its power to contract. This is referred to as *ventricular hypertrophy.* In addition, the ventricular chambers may dilate to accommodate those situations where there is an increased return of blood to the heart. The heart rate may speed up temporarily to increase the cardiac output.

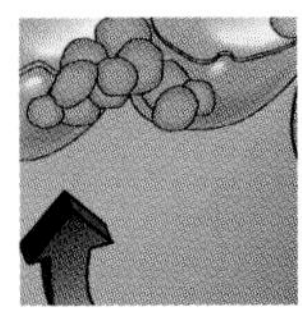

The manifestations of congestive heart failure vary depending on the nature of the stress and the heart's response, as well as which ventricle is involved. The left ventricle most commonly fails before the right because it is the major pumping chamber and is more exposed to factors underlying congestive heart failure than is the right ventricle. Eventually, however, both ventricles fail and the patient has signs and symptoms reflecting this.

In left ventricular failure, there is congestion that is caused by accumulation of fluid in the pulmonary circulation. The congestion interferes with breathing, and shortness of breath, a condition called *dyspnea*, is the result; usually the patient complains of fatigue without any exertion. *Orthopnea* occurs when the patient has difficulty breathing while lying down. The patient will often be forced to assume a propped up or sitting position in order to breathe comfortably. At times, the patient will be awakened during the night by shortness of breath and the sensation of suffocation and not getting enough air. This symptom is referred to as *paroxysmal nocturnal dyspnea.*

In right ventricular congestive heart failure, *edema* or swelling results when there is an accumulation of fluid in many of the organs and tissues. The liver becomes enlarged and tender because of fluid accumulation. It is most evident in the lower extremities, for example, as swollen ankles and feet.

The diagnosis of congestive heart failure is usually not difficult. A history of shortness of breath and edema is classic. Auscultation of the lungs reveals characteristic abnormal sounds, or *rales,* caused by congestion. The heart is usually enlarged and frequently there are abnormal heart sounds referred to as *gallop rhythms.* The presence of an enlarged, tender liver and edema of the lower extremities are also characteristic physical examination findings in congestive heart failure. In most instances, the physician will be able to identify the underlying cause of the condition. Arteriosclerotic heart disease, hypertension, and valvular disease are the most commonly encountered causes of congestive heart failure.

In treating congestive heart failure, the physician aims at two main goals. The first goal is to identify and, if possible, correct the underlying cause of congestive heart failure. A prime example of this would be diagnosis of a diseased aortic valve with subsequent surgical correction. Another example would be the successful treatment of hypertension with a combination of diet, drugs, and stress reduction. The second goal is to treat the congestive heart failure. The physician has a number of options in this regard. Salt (sodium) plays an important role in the body's retention of fluid, and the physician may prescribe a low-salt diet. If obesity is a problem, a program of weight reduction would be desirable. Diuretics are medications that assist the kidney in the regulation of body fluid balance, and they are commonly employed as treatment for congestive heart failure. Other pharmacologic agents are available that act directly on the heart to aid its contractility or control abnormal rhythms.

Most patients respond to the prescribed program, maintaining for many years a satisfactory condition with medication and with periodic checkups by the physician. In extreme cases where therapy has failed and the patient's life is in jeopardy, cardiac transplantation may be considered.

# Congestive Heart Failure

Congestive heart failure can affect the left or right ventricles, or both. The most common causes of congestive heart failure are diseased coronary arteries, high blood pressure, and diseases of the heart valves. Symptoms include shortness of breath (related to problems with blood circulation between the lungs and heart), swelling of legs and feet, and an enlarged and tender liver.

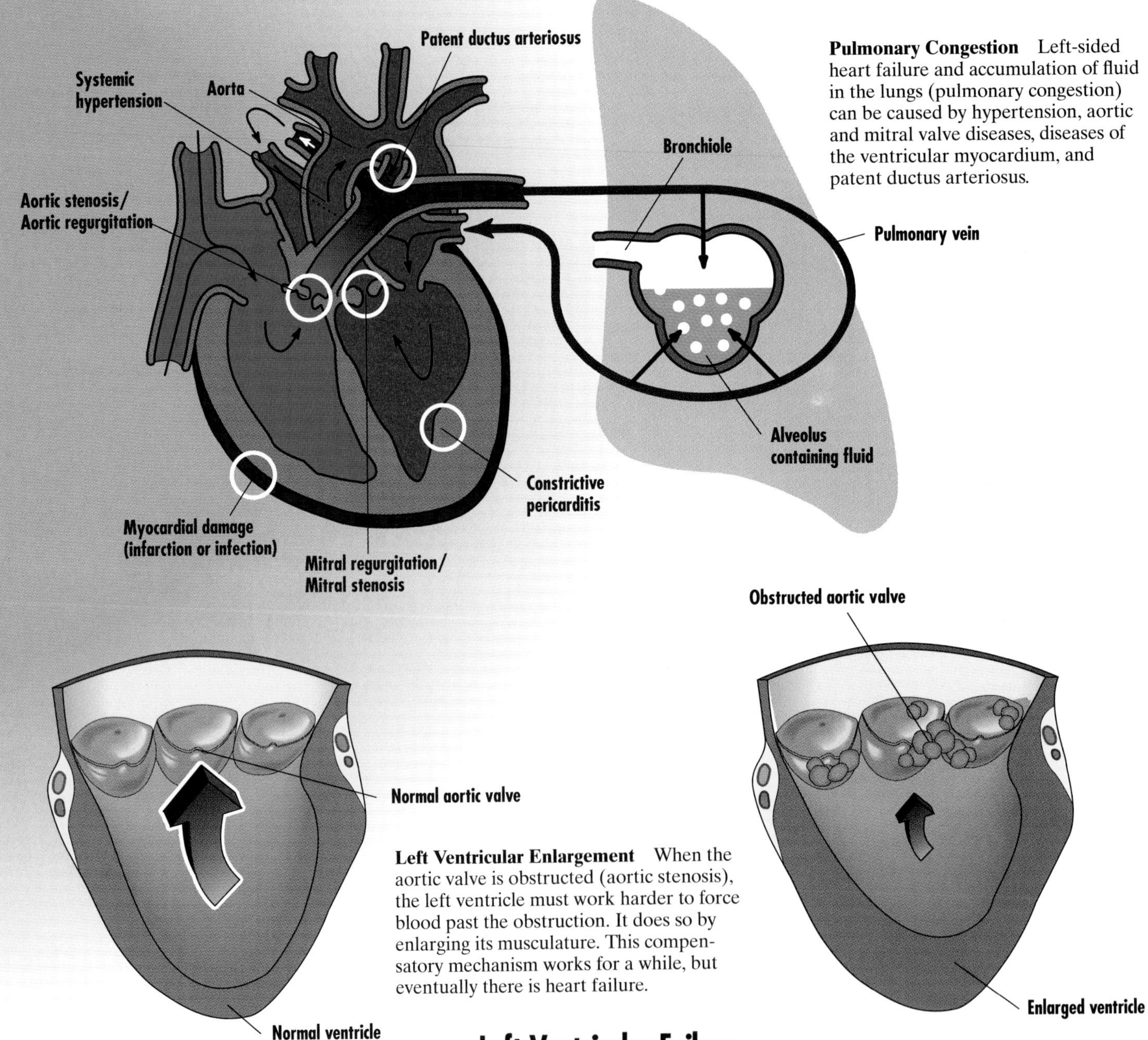


**Pulmonary Congestion** Left-sided heart failure and accumulation of fluid in the lungs (pulmonary congestion) can be caused by hypertension, aortic and mitral valve diseases, diseases of the ventricular myocardium, and patent ductus arteriosus.

**Left Ventricular Enlargement** When the aortic valve is obstructed (aortic stenosis), the left ventricle must work harder to force blood past the obstruction. It does so by enlarging its musculature. This compensatory mechanism works for a while, but eventually there is heart failure.

**Left Ventricular Failure**

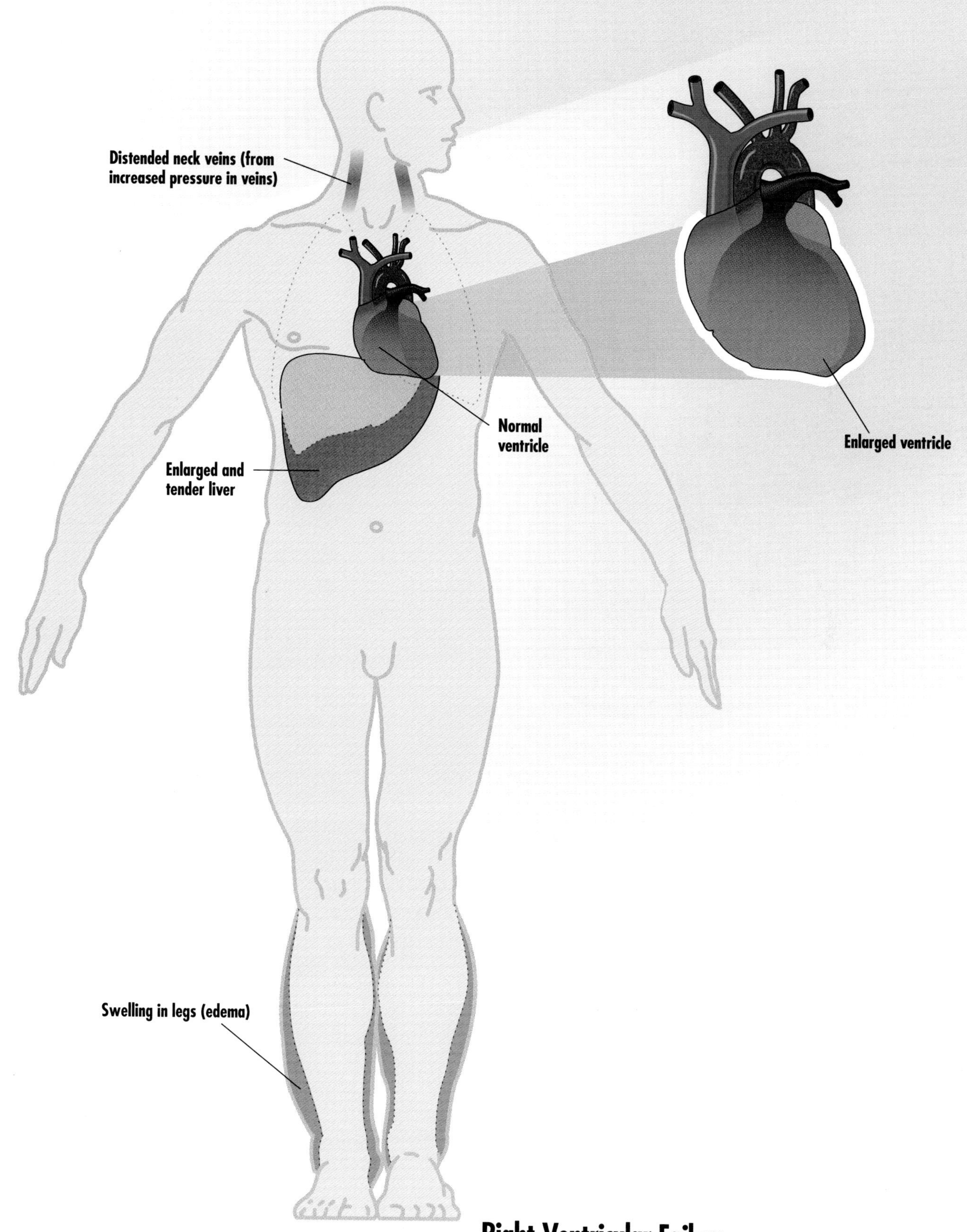


Right Ventricular Failure

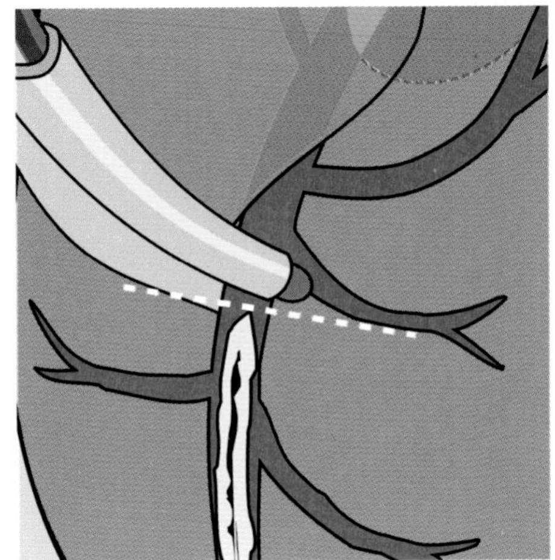

# Coronary Heart Disease

CORONARY HEART DISEASE is a term applied to a spectrum of heart diseases caused by partial or complete blockage, or occlusion, of one or more of the coronary arteries. Coronary heart disease produces ischemia, or deficiency of blood supply, of the myocardium. Thus, the term *ischemic heart disease* is used synonymously with coronary heart disease.

Coronary heart disease accounts for over 75% of all heart disease seen in the United States and is the most common cause of death in this country, accounting for over 500,000 deaths yearly. The incidence increases with age and is more common in men under the age of 45 than in women in that age group; however, by age 55, there is no difference in incidence between the sexes. It is the leading cause of death for men over the age of 35 and for both sexes over the age of 45.

The basic mechanism for the development of coronary heart disease is *atherosclerosis.* Atherosclerosis is one form of arteriosclerosis, which means thickening and hardening of the arterial walls. Atherosclerosis is characterized by the formation of *atheromas* on the inner lining, or intima, of arteries. An atheroma consists of a deposit or *plaque* of cholesterol, cholesterol by-products, fats, and blood-clotting elements. Eventually, the atheromas become calcified by the deposition of calcium and cause the artery to become hard and brittle. As the atheroma gradually enlarges, it increasingly impairs blood flow through the artery, and obstruction may be worsened by thrombus (clot) formation around the plaque. The tissue supplied by the vessel suffers *ischemia*, or lack of oxygen due to inadequate blood flow. If ischemia is brief, it may cause the characteristic anginal pain; if prolonged, it may cause *necrosis* (death) and scarring of tissue. Coronary heart disease involves the left ventricle almost exclusively, and ischemia of the left ventricle gives rise to the clinical manifestations of the disease.

Atherosclerosis may develop in any or all arteries, but there is a strong predilection for its development in the coronary arteries. The reasons for this are not understood, but we are aware of certain risk factors that predispose a person to coronary heart disease. There is, for example, a strong genetic factor; coronary heart disease tends to be inherited. Additional risk factors include male sex, advancing age, hypertension, diabetes, obesity, elevated blood cholesterol, smoking, and a sedentary lifestyle. An aggressive and competitive personality—the Type A personality—has been associated with coronary heart disease. Physical and emotional stress may play a contributing role in its development.

Fortunately, the coronary circulation is capable of forming new arteries, called *collaterals*, to meet the oxygen demands of the myocardium. Thus, if the reduction in blood flow and resultant ischemia occur gradually, the heart has time to form adequate secondary circulation. The patient, therefore, may have no symptoms or clinical findings.

When the atheromatous process occurs diffusely throughout the coronary circulation and collateral circulation is inadequate to satisfy the oxygen demands of the myocardium, the pumping action of the left ventricle may be impaired. This generalized process involving the myocardium is referred to as *atherosclerotic heart disease.* The result is "decompensation" of the left ventricle, that is, an inability of the left ventricle to maintain an adequate blood flow to the arteries.

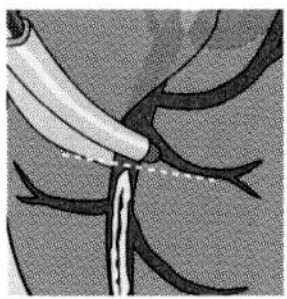

Atheromatous disease may develop such that myocardial oxygen demand is greater than myocardial blood flow, and the patient may experience *angina pectoris*—literally, pain in the chest. Transient ischemia of the myocardium is associated with the symptom of angina pectoris. Typically, angina pectoris is caused by physical exertion or emotional distress; cold weather and heavy meals are also precipitating factors. The predominant symptom is chest pain localized beneath the breast bone, or sternum, and described as squeezing or pressing. The pain may extend to the left shoulder and down the left arm or up into the neck and jaw. The pain is frequently accompanied by weakness, nausea, sweating, and apprehension. The pain usually disappears within a few minutes after the removal or discontinuation of the causative factor and is relieved by rest. Nitroglycerin is a medication that causes the blood vessels to dilate and thus increases blood flow. Taken under the tongue, nitroglycerin is effective in relieving the pain of angina pectoris. Many patients with this disease carry nitroglycerin with them for emergency use or in anticipation of conditions that typically may provoke an angina attack.

Given a typical history of angina pectoris, the physician usually has no difficulty in making a diagnosis. The physical examination, laboratory tests, and even the electrocardiogram may be normal when the patient is not experiencing symptoms. A normal electrocardiogram does not rule out ischemic heart disease, and the test most widely used in establishing the diagnosis is the exercise stress test. Performed with careful monitoring of the patient and with a physician present, the test is stopped immediately upon evidence of chest discomfort, shortness of breath, dizziness, blood pressure drop, or certain electrocardiographic changes. The stress test may be combined with a radioactive scan of the heart to determine the extent and region of the myocardial ischemia. If these tests are positive, the extent and sites of the coronary artery disease, as well as the functional effects on the left ventricle, may be determined by coronary arteriography or left heart catheterization.

Once the diagnosis of ischemic heart disease and angina pectoris is established, a decision is necessary concerning whether future treatment will be medical or surgical. Unless the patient is incapacitated by symptoms or the coronary arteriography shows advanced disease, a course of medical therapy is usually the first approach. Risk factors such as hypertension, diabetes, obesity, and elevated levels of blood cholesterol should be treated. Changes in diet, elimination of smoking, and modifications in lifestyle are frequently necessary. A careful program of exercise should be instituted. Pharmacologic treatment relies on nitrates such as nitroglycerin, which dilates blood vessels; beta-blockers, which reduce myocardial oxygen demand; and calcium-channel blockers, which dilate coronary arteries. Long-acting derivatives of nitroglycerin that are taken orally, or by patch or paste, are also available for long-term prevention of attacks, and may be used in conjunction with nitroglycerin taken under the tongue.

The decision for surgical therapy rests on the clinical history, stress test results, and coronary arteriography findings. Patients may be considered surgical candidates if angina symptoms are very severe and medical therapy ineffective, if the stress test is markedly positive with minimal exercise, or if arteriography shows either disease involving three coronary arteries or over 50% narrowing of a major coronary artery. Several effective procedures are available. Coronary artery bypass surgery uses a vein graft to bypass the coronary artery obstruction. Cardiopulmonary bypass (heart-lung machine) makes surgery possible with the heart under direct vision. All venous blood is directed to an oxygenator outside the body and is then pumped back into an artery. Cannulas (large catheters) are placed in both the superior and inferior venae cavae, and the venous blood is directed to an oxygenator that removes the carbon dioxide and replaces it with oxygen. A pump then directs the blood back into the body by a cannula placed in a femoral artery in the groin. An alternative procedure, *angioplasty*, or balloon dilation, of the constricted artery, is much less complex and incapacitating than is bypass surgery. Surgical removal of the actual atheromatous obstruction, a procedure called endarterectomy, is another approach.

An *acute myocardial infarction* occurs if there is complete obstruction of a coronary artery, usually due to a clot adjacent to an atherosclerotic plaque. In other words, the area of myocardium normally supplied with oxygenated blood by the involved artery is completely deprived of blood. The result is a myocardial infarction, an area of myocardium that is essentially dead and cannot function. The consequences of an acute myocardial infarction depend on both the location of the vessel and the exact area of the myocardium involved. If the area of infarction is large or particularly critical, effective pumping action of the entire left ventricle ceases, cardiac output drops, and unless emergency therapy is successful, death is the result.

Regardless of size, any myocardial infarction is dangerous because it may interfere with effective pumping action of the heart or with effective electrical conduction within the heart, thus causing serious ventricular arrhythmias. Arrhythmias are in turn life-threatening if they prevent effective ventricular pumping action.

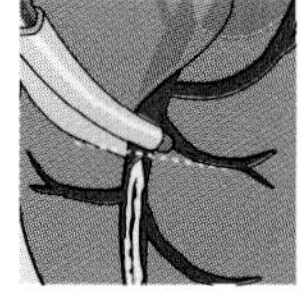

Small myocardial infarctions may go unnoticed if the area of myocardial involvement is small and the total damage to the heart is minimal. These are referred to as *silent myocardial infarctions.* Their presence is not often detected until an electrocardiogram is taken for another purpose.

In typical myocardial infarction, the patient has severe and unrelenting chest pain, usually characterized as crushing or pressing, and localized beneath the breast bone, often radiating to the left shoulder and arm or into the neck and jaws. The pain is accompanied by sweating, nausea, and weakness and is not relieved by nitroglycerin.

The electrocardiogram is critical in the diagnosis of an acute myocardial infarction. Except in extremely rare cases, characteristic changes are seen immediately and the electrocardiogram progresses through a series of changes thereafter. The electrocardiogram leads help to establish the anatomic location of the infarct. Posterior (back), anterior (front), inferior (low), and lateral (side) are common myocardial sites for infarction. The anatomic locations may overlap; for example, an anterolateral infarct indicates an infarct involving both the anterior and lateral walls of the left ventricle.

The laboratory is also of value in the diagnosis of an acute myocardial infarction. The myocardium contains particular muscle enzymes that are released from the damaged tissue into the blood where they can be measured. The most sensitive and specific of these enzymes is creatine-phosphokinase (CPK). Blood levels of CPK rise to high levels after a myocardial infarction.

Patients with a demonstrable or suspected myocardial infarction should be hospitalized, preferably in a coronary intensive care unit. These units are designed and equipped for continuous monitoring of the patient's vital signs and electrocardiogram. If there is danger of congestive heart failure, the patient's venous pressure can also be monitored.

Acute therapy for a myocardial infarction includes pain relief, sedation, and oxygen. Medications have recently been introduced that, if administered promptly after the onset of symptoms, can promote dissolution of the obstructing thrombus in the coronary artery, thereby reducing the extent of damage to the heart. Most patients with an acute myocardial infarction are placed on anticoagulant (blood thinner) medication designed to protect against the development of clots (thrombi) on the inner wall of the ventricle at the site of the infarction. Thrombi are dangerous because they tend to break apart and send pieces, or emboli, to other areas of the body. Anticoagulants may be prescribed indefinitely to prevent this complication.

If several days elapse without complications, the patient is allowed to increase his or her activities, and after about one week can be discharged to convalesce at home. Rigorous treatment of risk factors, if present, should be continued indefinitely, as it has been demonstrated to be effective in the prevention of future myocardial infarctions.

Most patients do well after recovery from an acute myocardial infarction. Collateral circulation helps the injured myocardium return to function, although fully normal pumping action may never be possible. The electrocardiogram will usually manifest evidence of residual damage from any infarction. Proper treatment and elimination of risk factors remain a life-long necessity.

# Coronary Heart Disease

### *Coronary Heart Disease Risk Factors*

- Genetics
- Advancing Age
- Hypertension
- Diabetes
- Obesity
- High Cholesterol Level
- Smoking
- Lack of Exercise
- Type A Personality
- Stress

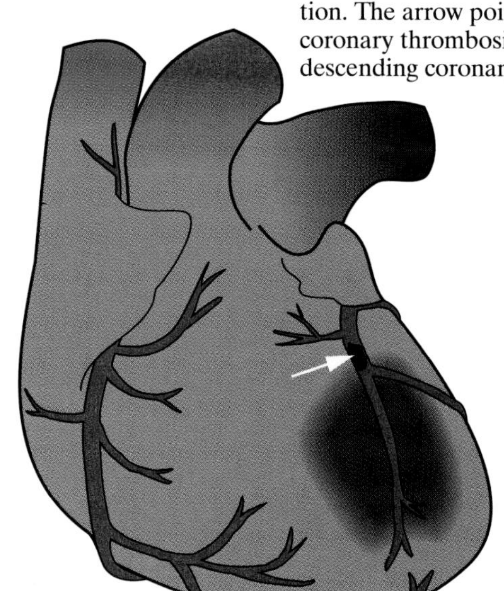

**Myocardial Infarction** The illustration shows an anterior wall myocardial infarction. The arrow points to an occlusion, or coronary thrombosis, in the left anterior descending coronary artery.

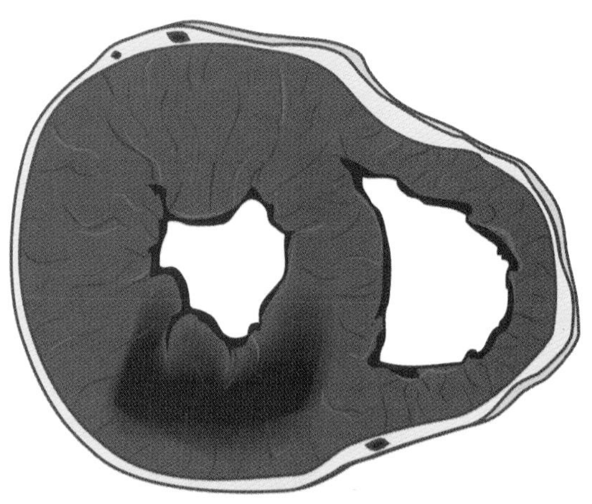

**Cross-section of the Heart** The dark red area represents an acute myocardial infarction of the left ventricular posterior wall.

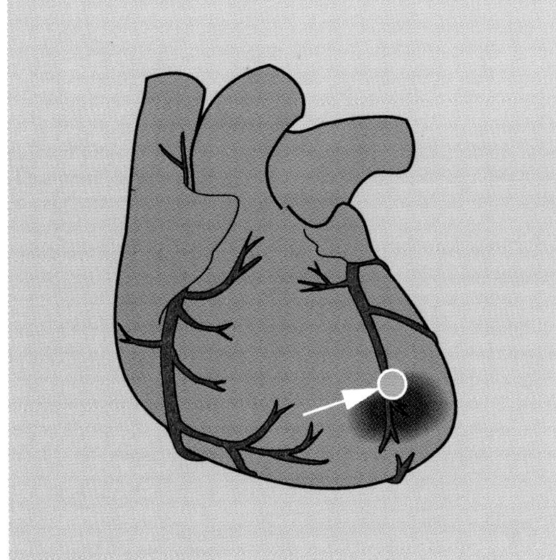

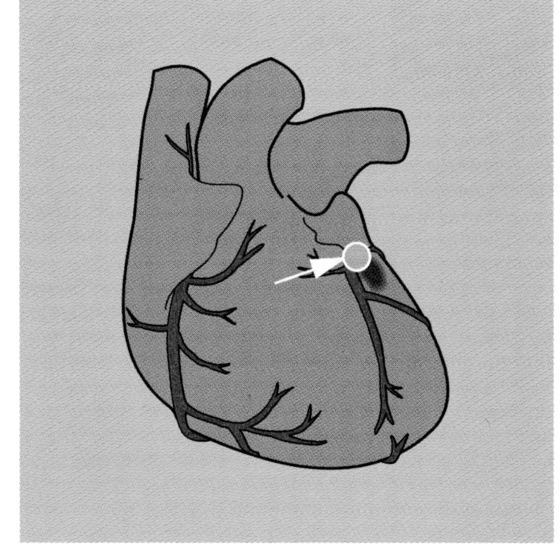

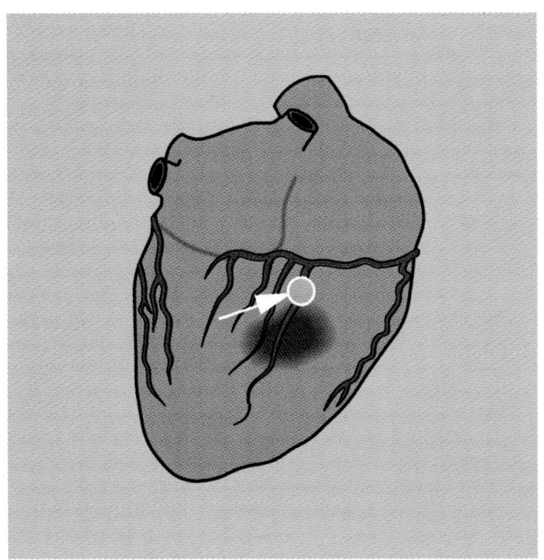

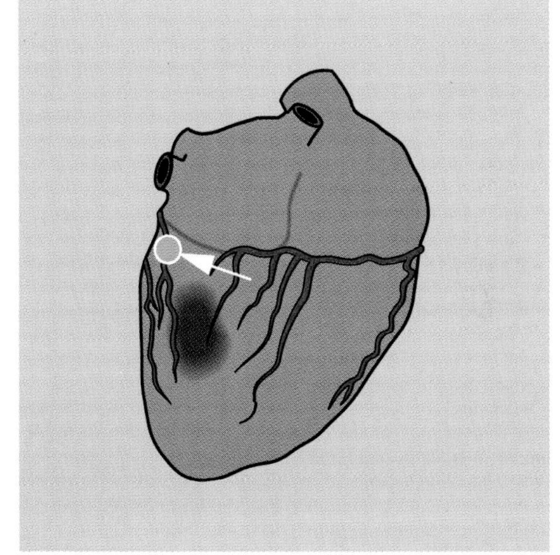

**Potential Myocardial Infarction Sites** Locations of myocardial infarctions on the anterior (top) and posterior (above) walls of the left ventricle secondary to obstructions of the branches of the major coronary arteries. The exact location of the infarction depends on the coronary artery branch that is occluded. Occlusion of the major coronary arteries results in larger areas of infarction.

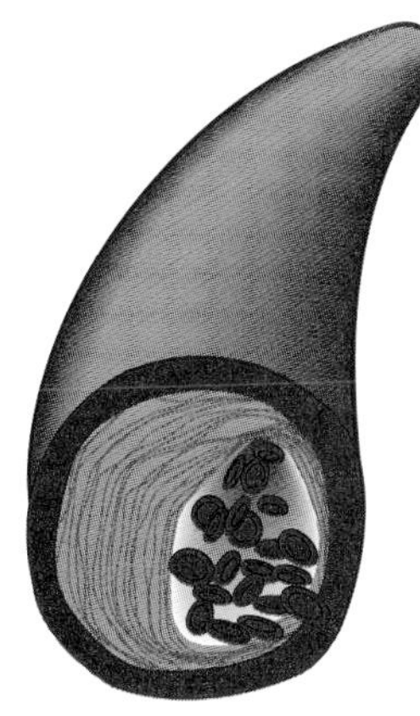

**Coronary Artery Blockage** On the left is a cross-section view of partial blockage (occlusion) of the artery by an atheroma. This degree of obstruction involving a large coronary artery could produce angina pectoris. The cross-section on the right shows complete obstruction of the artery by an atheroma and superimposed thrombosis, or blood clot. This could lead to myocardial infarction.

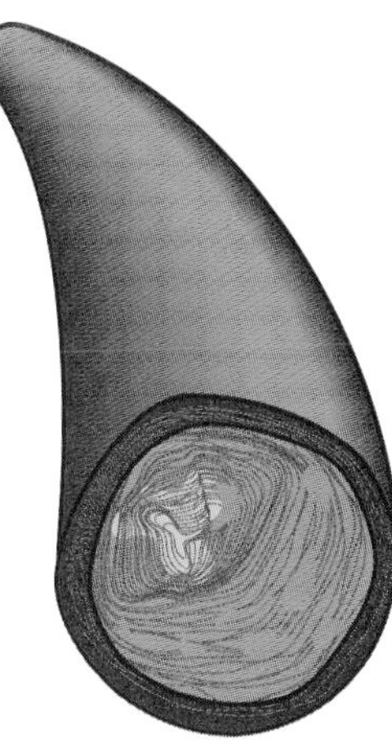

# Treatment of Coronary Heart Disease

Coronary heart disease can be treated either with medicines or surgically. The decision of which therapy to use depends on many factors, but among them are degree of incapacitation of the patient, clinical history, and stress test and coronary arteriography results. Medical treatment often includes medications that dilate blood vessels (nitrates, such as nitroglycerin), reduce myocardial oxygen demand (beta-blockers), and dilate coronary arteries (calcium-channel blockers). Surgical treatment includes coronary bypass, angioplasty, and endarterectomy. Regardless of whether the treatment is medical or surgical, risk factors such as high blood pressure, smoking, and obesity must be addressed if treatment is to be completely successful.

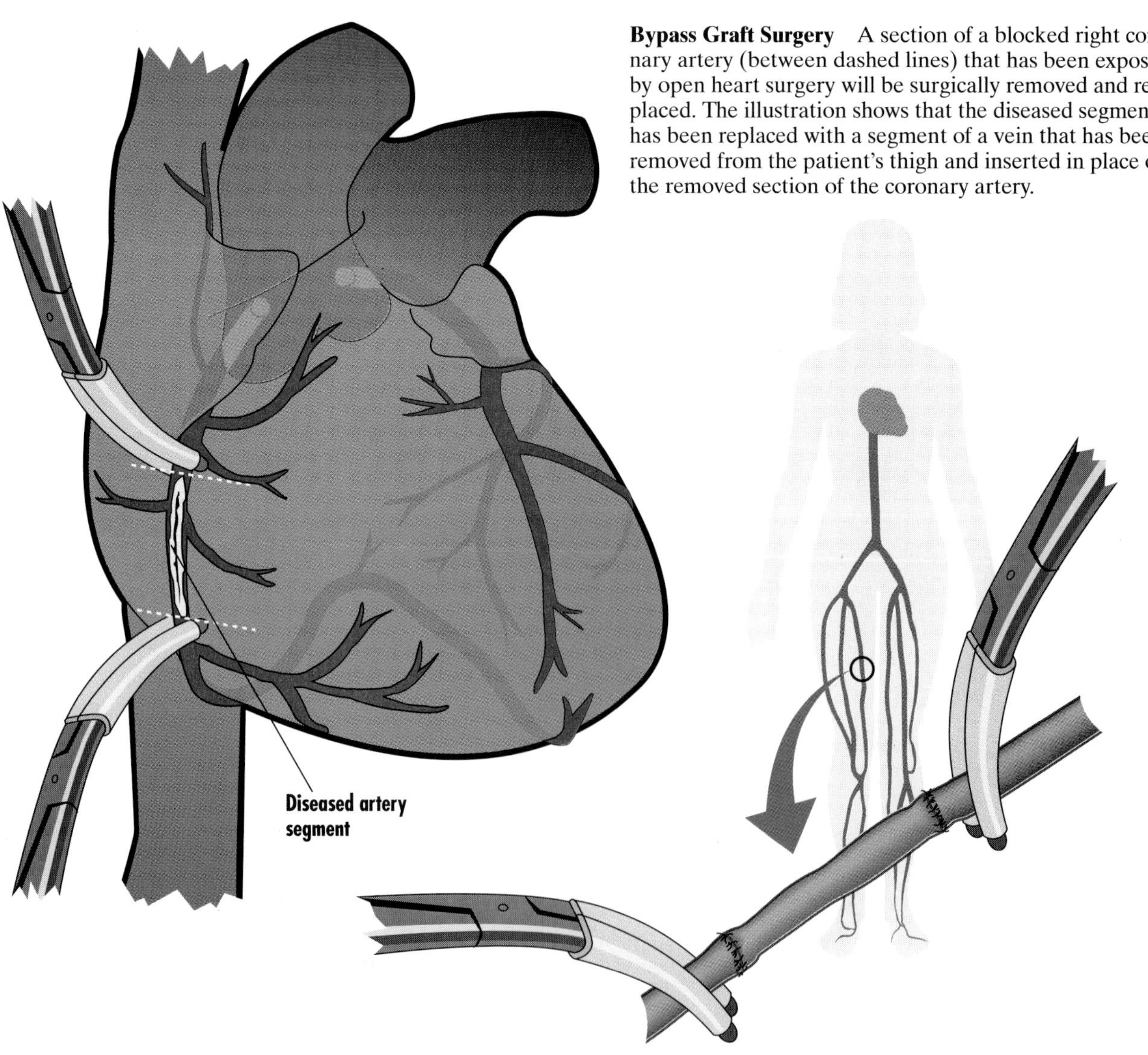


**Bypass Graft Surgery** A section of a blocked right coronary artery (between dashed lines) that has been exposed by open heart surgery will be surgically removed and replaced. The illustration shows that the diseased segment has been replaced with a segment of a vein that has been removed from the patient's thigh and inserted in place of the removed section of the coronary artery.

**Cardiopulmonary Bypass (Heart-Lung Machine)** A heart-lung machine enables heart surgery to be performed while the surgeon directly observes the heart. Tubes (called cannulas) are placed in the inferior and superior venae cavae, diverting all venous blood to an oxygenator that removes the carbon dioxide and replaces the oxygen. The oxygenated blood is then pumped into an artery, usually the femoral artery in the groin. In some instances, the venous cannula is placed in the right atrium.

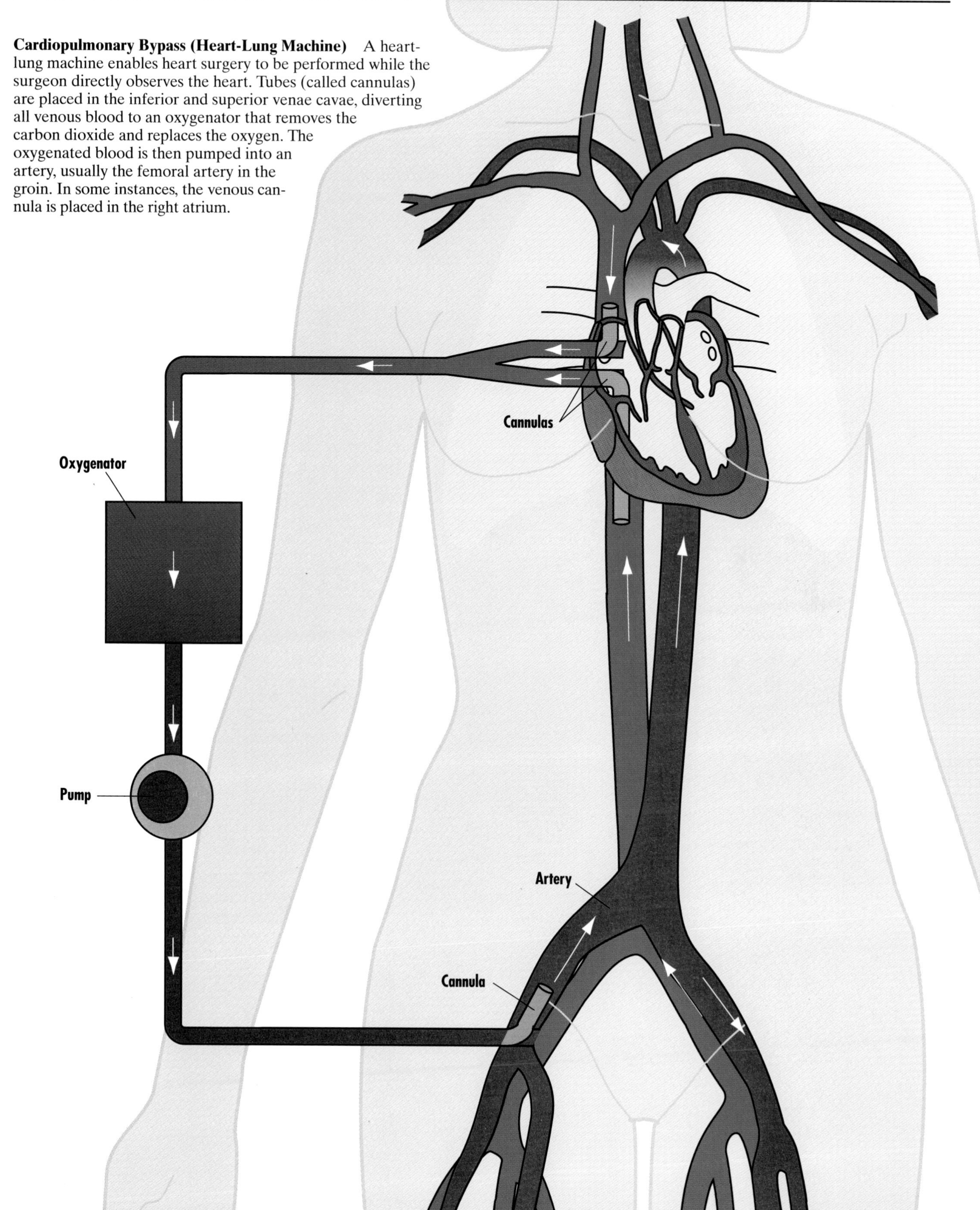

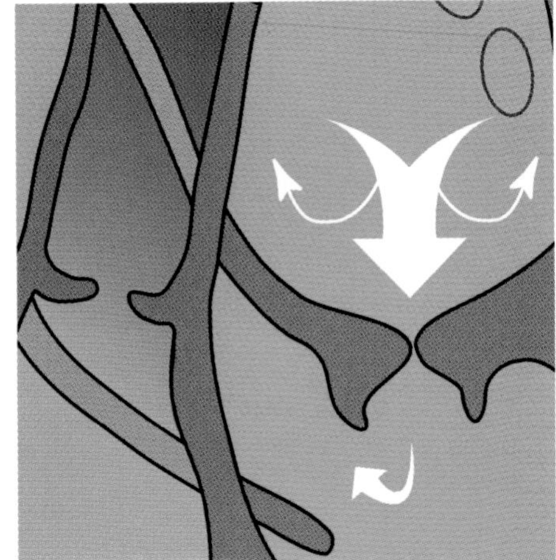

# Valvular Heart Disease

DEFECTS OF THE heart valves may be of congenital or acquired origin. Whatever the cause, a defective valve places an unnatural strain on the heart that, without treatment, ultimately results in heart failure. There are two general types of valve defect—*stenosis* and *regurgitation.* In valvular stenosis, the opening of the valve is smaller than normal and the aperture through which blood flows from a heart chamber is narrowed. In valvular regurgitation, there is widening of the valve aperture or impairment of valve closure, with resultant backflow or regurgitation of blood into the heart chamber from which it has been ejected. Stenosis is usually accompanied by some degree of regurgitation.

Each of the four heart valves—the mitral and aortic on the left side of the heart, and the tricuspid and pulmonic on the right side of the heart—may be involved individually or in any combination. Defects of the tricuspid and pulmonic valves are usually of congenital origin and may be found with other congenital abnormalities of the heart. These defects are rarely of acquired origin.

Rheumatic fever is the most common cause of acquired mitral and aortic valve disease. The acute episode of rheumatic fever usually occurs in childhood between the ages of 5 and 15, but the valve consequences do not become evident until 10 to 15 years later. The incidence of acute rheumatic fever following a streptococcal infection is less than 3%. However, about 65% of patients with rheumatic fever will eventually develop valvular heart disease. Unrecognized forms of the disease often occur, and about half of the patients with rheumatic valvular involvement have no history of prior rheumatic fever. Rheumatic fever will be discussed in detail later in the book.

The valve most frequently involved in rheumatic heart disease is the mitral valve. Next in frequency is a combination of mitral and aortic valve disease, and finally, aortic valve disease alone. The tricuspid and pulmonic valves are rarely involved.

In *mitral regurgitation*, there is increased pressure in the left atrium because the valve does not close properly and there is regurgitation of blood into the left atrium during left ventricular systole. The left atrium may become huge as a result of this condition. The increased pressure and volume in the left atrium cause increased pressure and an accumulation of fluid (congestion) in the pulmonary circulation. The patient experiences shortness of breath (dyspnea). Fatigue is another common complaint and is caused by reduced cardiac output that occurs as a consequence of the large volume of blood being regurgitated into the left atrium. The heart must compensate for the decreased cardiac output and maintain arterial blood pressure, so the left ventricle increases its size (dilates) and its muscle mass (hypertrophies) to increase its stroke volume. Mitral regurgitation may be well tolerated for many years, but eventually the pumping mechanism fails because of the increased work load. When this occurs, and the patient does not respond satisfactorily to medical treatment, surgical treatment becomes necessary.

The surgical treatment of mitral regurgitation is replacement of the valve with a prosthetic valve or one of porcine (pig) origin. The risks of surgery rise proportionately to the degree of decreased left ventricular function. The patient, therefore, is treated medically until his or her condition is optimal for surgical intervention. Lifelong use of anticoagulant (blood thinning) medication to prevent clot formation on a prosthetic valve is necessary for these patients.

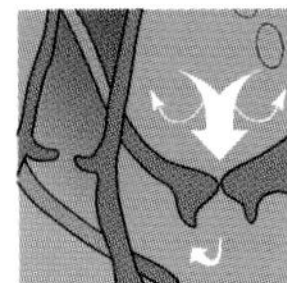

*Mitral valve prolapse*, a fairly common condition, is seen primarily in women under the age of 40. Chest pain, fatigue, and arrhythmias felt as palpitations are common clinical findings. Varying degrees of mitral regurgitation may be noted. The leaflets of the mitral valve, abnormally large and floppy, bulge into the atrium on left ventricular contraction, producing a systolic murmur preceded by a characteristic clicking sound. The echocardiogram is useful in making the diagnosis and determining the degree of mitral regurgitation. Mitral valve prolapse generally requires no treatment, although the patient may be cautioned and periodically checked for the development of arrhythmias.

*Mitral stenosis* is a narrowing of the valve opening that results from scarring and thickening of the valve leaflets as a consequence of rheumatic fever. Flow from the left atrium to the left ventricle is impeded by the small valve aperture. As the obstruction progresses, pressure in the left atrium increases and is transmitted to the pulmonary veins. As a consequence, the patient's first symptoms may be dyspnea or orthopnea, at times along with production of bloody sputum. As the left atrium becomes enlarged, and the flow of blood sluggish, clots (thrombi) may form in its cavity. If these clots detach and move through the systemic circulation to other organs as *emboli,* they may damage the circulation and function of that organ. Long-term anticoagulant medication is prescribed to prevent emboli. *Atrial fibrillation*, an arrhythmia, is a common complication of mitral stenosis due to the enlarged left atrium. As pulmonary hypertension and congestion progress, there may be congestive heart failure of the right ventricle.

Characteristic findings from the physical examination usually enable the physician to make the diagnosis of mitral stenosis. The principal diagnostic finding is a characteristic murmur that mitral stenosis produces. Certain radiographic and electrocardiographic features produced by the large left atrium in mitral stenosis cases are also helpful in making the diagnosis. The diagnosis can be confirmed by echocardiography; if surgery is planned, the degree of stenosis can be determined by cardiac catheterization. In patients who have symptoms, surgical replacement of the mitral valve is the treatment of choice. Before surgery, medical therapy aims to correct congestive heart failure and control arrhythmias.

When seen as an isolated defect, *aortic stenosis* is commonly a congenital heart abnormality, a bicuspid, or two-leaflet valve; if it occurs as a result of rheumatic fever, it is often accompanied by mitral valve disease. The aortic cusps become thickened and irregular, with gradual narrowing of the opening between the left ventricle and the aorta. As a result, the left ventricle has to work against increased resistance to maintain cardiac output. The muscle mass of the left ventricle enlarges to perform this greater work load, but eventually there is pump failure, which leads to congestive heart failure.

A characteristic harsh murmur during systole caused by the flow of blood through the narrow, irregular valve opening makes the diagnosis. The deformity of the aortic valve causes excessive myocardial oxygen demand, which may make the patient symptomatic with angina. Cardiac catheterization and coronary angiography should be performed to assess the degree of stenosis and the adequacy of the coronary circulation. Surgical replacement with a prosthetic or porcine valve is the treatment of choice. Prosthetic valve replacement requires lifelong anticoagulant treatment.

*Aortic regurgitation* may result from rheumatic fever or occur secondary to conditions that either cause the aorta to dilate or prevent normal aortic valve closure. Most common causes include syphilis, certain congenital disorders, and diseases of the aorta itself. Rheumatic fever causes thickening and shortening of the cusp margins so that the cusps do not meet tightly. Aortic stenosis is often accompanied by some degree of regurgitation.

Aortic regurgitation allows a backflow of blood from the aorta into the left ventricle during diastole, when the left atrium is normally draining into the left ventricle. The result is an excessive volume of blood for the left ventricle. The ventricle's pumping work is magnified by this increased load and the muscle hypertrophies to meet the corresponding demands. The huge left ventricle eventually decompensates and congestive heart failure ensues.

The regurgitant flow from the aorta creates a blowing murmur—a murmur that sounds like a blowing noise, soft and smooth—during diastole. Because the aortic valve fails to close completely, the diastolic pressure is low. Low diastolic pressure coupled with high systolic pressure created by the overworked left ventricle causes a wide pulse pressure, that is, a much larger than normal difference between the systolic and diastolic pressures. This is manifested in bounding pulses, with brisk upstroke and rapid falloff. Increasing heart size and the development of left ventricular failure are indications for surgical replacement of the diseased valve. As with aortic stenosis, prosthetic or porcine replacements may be used.

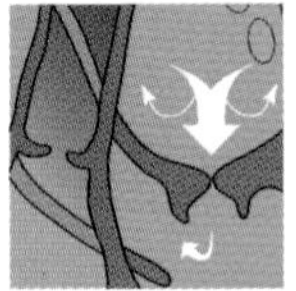

# Defects of the Heart Valves

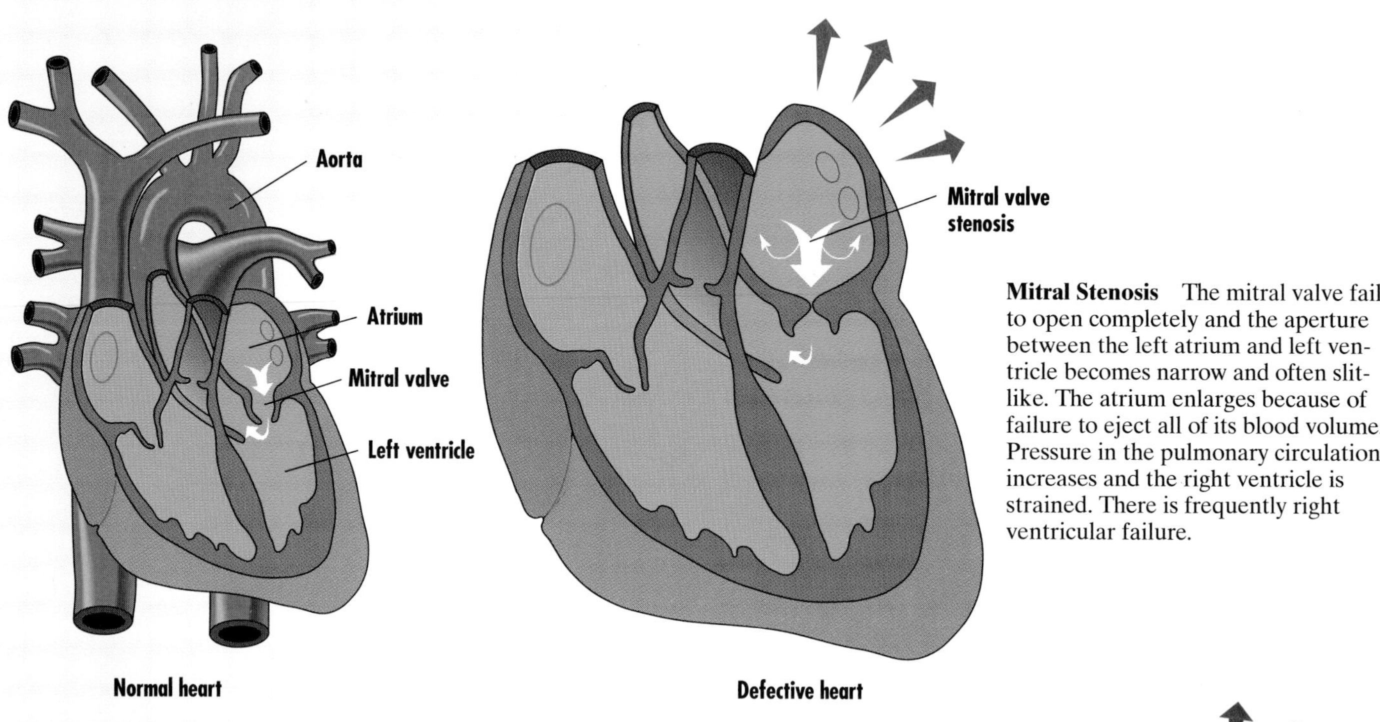


Normal heart

Defective heart

**Mitral Stenosis** The mitral valve fails to open completely and the aperture between the left atrium and left ventricle becomes narrow and often slit-like. The atrium enlarges because of failure to eject all of its blood volume. Pressure in the pulmonary circulation increases and the right ventricle is strained. There is frequently right ventricular failure.

**Mitral Regurgitation** The mitral valve remains partly open during left ventricular contraction, allowing regurgitation of blood back into the left atrium. The left atrium becomes enlarged, and pressure and volume increase within its chamber. This, in turn, increases pressure and volume in the pulmonary circulation, resulting in the patient experiencing shortness of breath. Eventually, the right ventricle fails in working against increased pulmonary circulation resistance, and there is right-sided congestive heart failure.

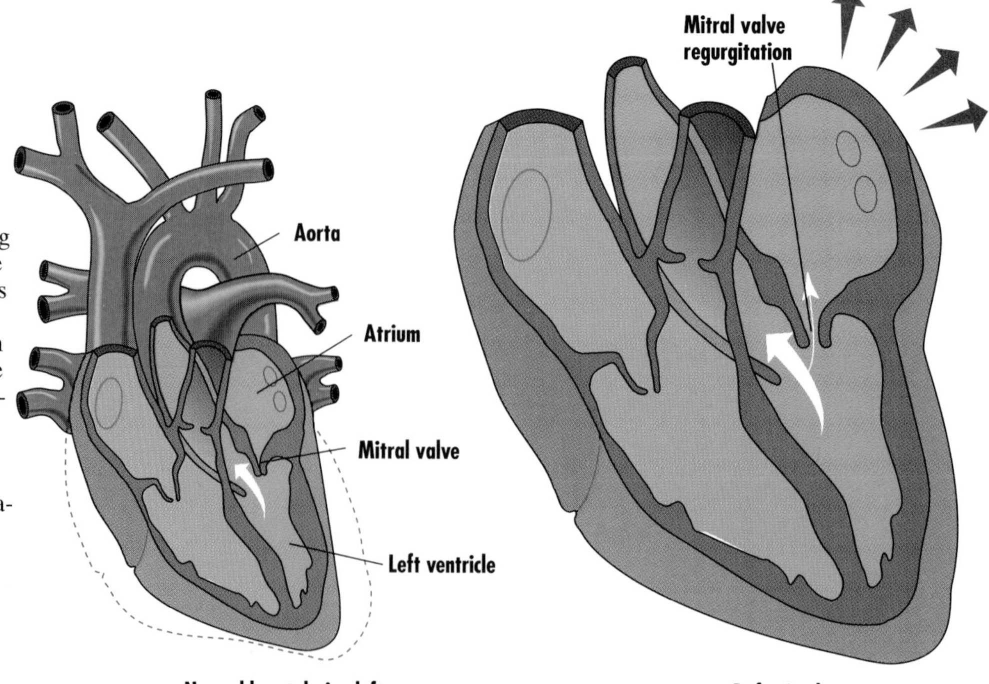


Normal heart during left ventricular contraction

Defective heart

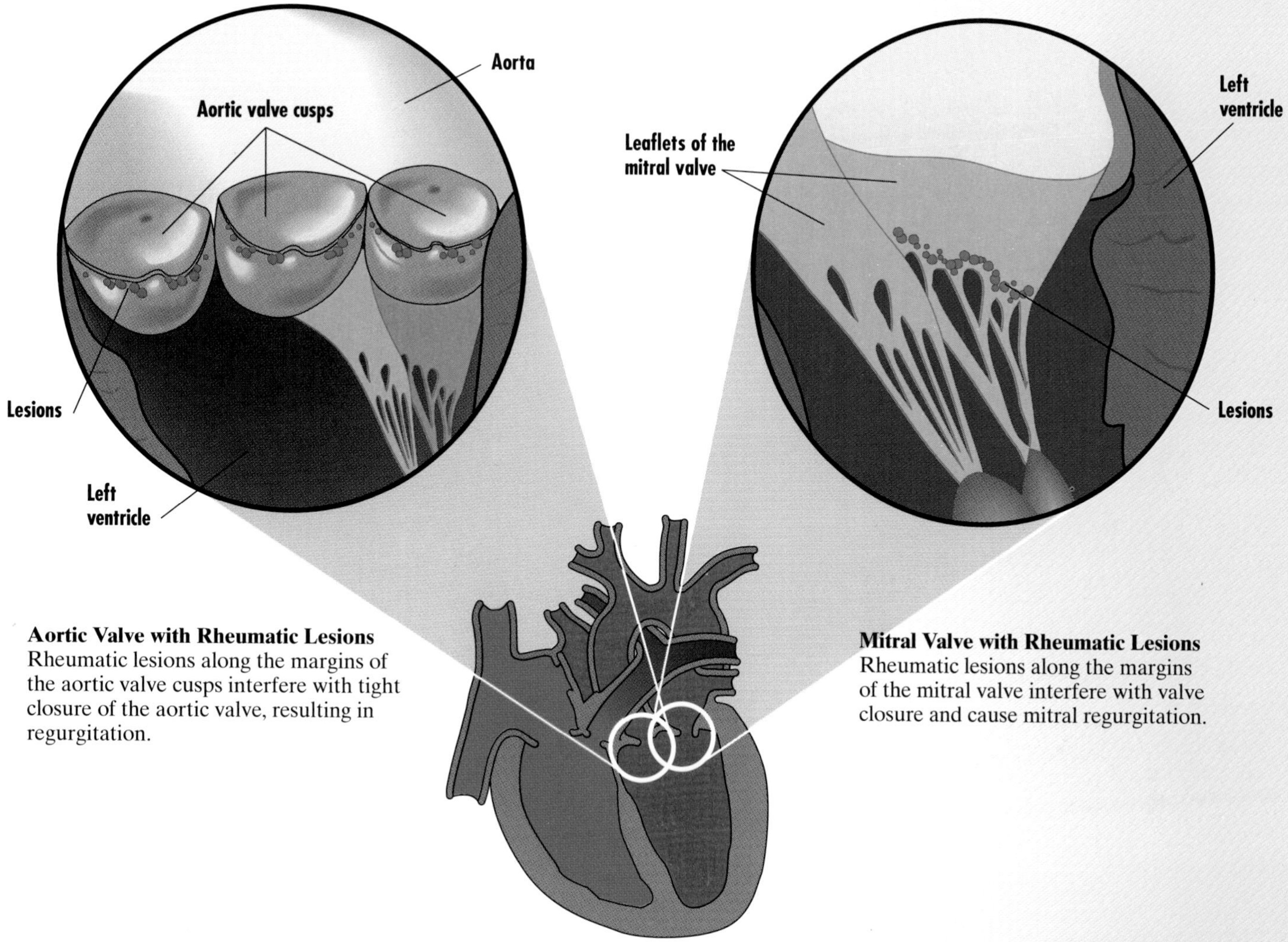

Aorta

Aortic valve cusps

Lesions

Left ventricle

Leaflets of the mitral valve

Left ventricle

Lesions

**Aortic Valve with Rheumatic Lesions** Rheumatic lesions along the margins of the aortic valve cusps interfere with tight closure of the aortic valve, resulting in regurgitation.

**Mitral Valve with Rheumatic Lesions** Rheumatic lesions along the margins of the mitral valve interfere with valve closure and cause mitral regurgitation.

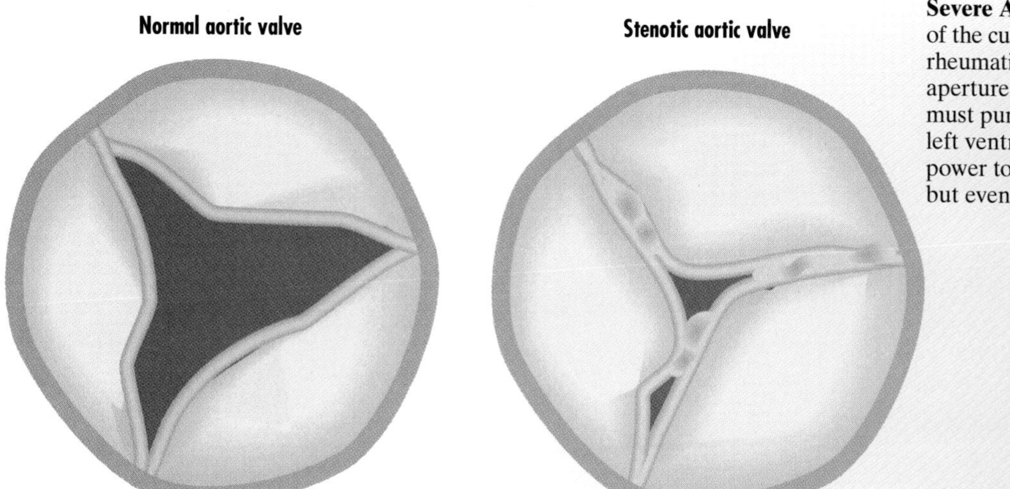


**Severe Aortic Stenosis** The margins of the cusps have fused as a result of rheumatic fever. There is now a narrow aperture through which the left ventricle must pump blood into the aorta. The left ventricle increases in size and power to overcome this obstruction, but eventually fails.

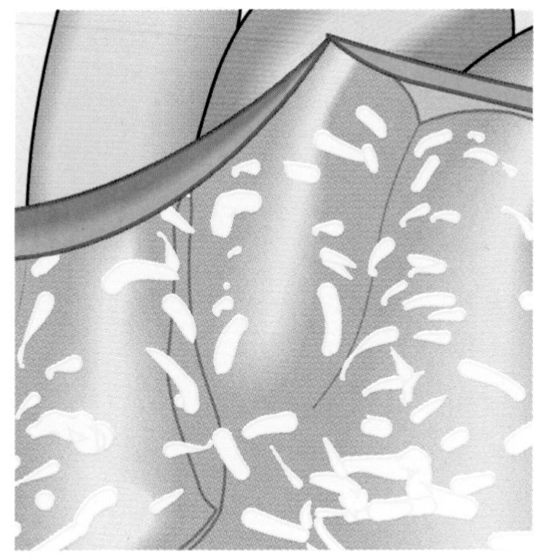

# Infections of the Heart

THE HEART MAY be one of several or the sole organ affected by an infection. The infectious agent may be a bacterium, virus, fungus, or parasite; or an inflammation symptomatically similar to infection may be part of an allergic or hypersensitivity reaction. Any one or any combination of the three layers of the heart may be involved. In *pericarditis,* the thin, fibrous membrane surrounding the heart is infected; in *myocarditis,* the cardiac muscle is involved; and in *endocarditis,* there is an infection of the inner lining of the heart chambers and valves.

*Rheumatic fever* is the most common and most important disease in this group. There is convincing evidence that rheumatic fever is caused by a certain type of *streptococcus* (group A), and usually occurs after an infection of the throat. Rheumatic fever is not due to direct action by the streptococcus, but results from an interaction between toxins produced by the bacteria, called *antigens,* and defense substances produced by the body in response to the infection, called *antibodies.* Rheumatic fever is an example of what is referred to as an *antigen-antibody reaction.* Actually, rheumatic fever develops in less than 3% of streptococcus group A infections. Recent studies suggest that there may be a genetically determined susceptibility to acute rheumatic fever.

Rheumatic fever may occur at any age, but is most commonly seen in children between the ages of 5 and 15. The disease is characterized by fever and painful and swollen joints and often by a variety of skin rashes. An acute inflammation of the heart, *carditis,* accompanies these symptoms and is manifested by pericarditis, myocarditis, and endocarditis. Cardiac changes may be detected by the physician as murmurs or arrhythmias on physical examination of the patient, or as abnormalities on the electrocardiogram, and the diagnosis is suggested by certain laboratory tests.

The severity of rheumatic fever varies from trivial to extremely serious, and death may result. The duration of rheumatic fever also varies from days to months, and recurrence is common. Salicylates, or drugs related to aspirin, and corticosteroids, such as prednisone, are helpful in alleviating the acute symptoms. Unfortunately, about 65% of patients with acute rheumatic fever develop valvular heart disease, although it may take years for the valve defects to become apparent.

The incidence of rheumatic fever is decreasing in the U.S. because of the availability of antibiotics that are effective in treating the streptococcus. Therapy of acute streptococcal infections such as sore throat should be continued for 10 days to prevent recurrence and to assure destruction of the streptococcus. In about half of the cases of rheumatic valvular heart disease, a preceding streptococcal infection has not been recognized.

Patients with rheumatic heart disease are susceptible to infection superimposed on their damaged valves. This condition is called *subacute bacterial endocarditis* and is caused by infection of the damaged valves by types of streptococcus (other than group A) and by *enterococcus*, an organism commonly found in the gastrointestinal and urinary tracts. In many cases of subacute bacterial endocarditis, the source of the infection is not apparent; as streptococcus organisms are normally present in the mouth, they may invade the bloodstream following injuries as slight as tooth cleaning and brushing. Once in the bloodstream and circulating through organs, the bacteria may cause disease. For this reason, many patients with rheumatic heart disease are placed on preventive, or prophylactic, antibiotics indefinitely, and all must take antibiotics before dental procedures or surgery.

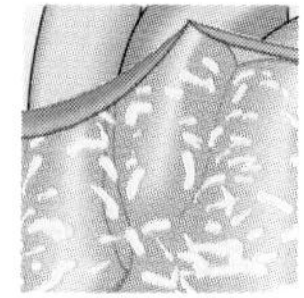

The diagnosis of subacute bacterial endocarditis is suspected when a patient with rheumatic heart disease develops fever and changes in the character of his or her heart murmurs. Organisms lodged on the damaged heart valves produce clusters or vegetations, pieces of which may dislodge and travel through the blood as *emboli.* Evidence of emboli may be seen on the skin or may cause damage to the brain, kidneys, or other organs.

The diagnosis of subacute bacterial endocarditis is established by isolating the offending bacterium in blood cultures. Treatment is use of an appropriate antibiotic, that is, one to which the bacterium is sensitive. High doses of antibiotic, usually given intravenously for a prolonged period of time, are usually necessary. The occurrence of subacute bacterial endocarditis may hasten the need for surgical valve replacement.

*Acute bacterial endocarditis* may occur on a normal endocardium or heart valve. It is frequently caused by the *staphylococcus* bacterium, but may be caused by any organism entering the bloodstream from any site of prior infection. In contrast to the slower process of subacute bacterial endocarditis, acute bacterial endocarditis is a rapid, devastating disease that causes fatality unless treated promptly and vigorously. The patient has a high fever, and rapid destruction of heart valves by the infectious process causes murmurs and congestive heart failure. Localized collections of infection, *abscesses,* may form in other organs such as the brain and kidneys. Treatment is with high doses of antibiotics to which the bacterium is sensitive. Permanent valve damage is a frequent complication for those patients who recover.

*Acute myocarditis* may also occur in rheumatic fever but more commonly is caused by viral agents. A mild, clinically insignificant form accompanies many viral diseases. Bacteria are rarely the cause of myocarditis. *Coxsackie virus*—so named for the town in New York where it was first identified—is the most common cause of acute myocarditis. The virus produces damage throughout the myocardium that may interfere with its pumping action. Congestive heart failure occurs only occasionally but may be life-threatening. There is no specific treatment for Coxsackie virus, but research is being conducted on the use of antiviral agents.

*Acute pericarditis* is the result of a variety of causes in addition to rheumatic fever. These causes include bacteria, viruses, fungi, parasites, allergic reactions, reactions to certain drugs, and penetrating injuries of the heart. Pericarditis frequently occurs in conjunction with an acute myocardial infarction or occurs as an immunologic reaction after cardiac surgery.

The most common symptom of acute pericarditis is sudden, sharp chest pain aggravated by breathing and by lying down. The pain tends to be relieved by the sitting position or by leaning forward. Fever may be present. The physician may hear a *pericardial friction rub* on auscultation of the heart. The hallmark rub is caused by friction between the inflamed pericardium and the contracting myocardium. Irregular or rapid pulse may be noted. There are also certain characteristic changes in the electrocardiogram that are actually caused by involvement of the underlying myocardium rather than being generated by the pericardium, which has no electrical activity.

Occasionally, there may be an accumulation of fluid within the pericardial sac, a condition called *pericardial effusion,* as a result of the pericarditis. Analysis of a sample of pericardial fluid obtained by needle aspiration provides valuable information that may indicate the cause of the underlying pericarditis and is helpful in planning appropriate therapy.

If the pericardial effusion increases to the point of restricting ventricular filling, it may produce *cardiac tamponade*. Accumulation of fluid within the inelastic pericardial sac may interfere with the venous inflow to the heart. The cardiac output falls, arterial blood pressure decreases, and shock may develop. Therapeutic drainage of the fluid is necessary under these conditions.

If pericarditis is recurrent or persists in a chronic fashion, *constrictive pericarditis* may result. When this happens, the pericardium becomes scarred, thickened, and adherent to the underlying myocardium. Calcium may be deposited in the diseased pericardium. Constrictive pericarditis interferes with the contractility of the heart and leads to heart failure, particularly of the right ventricle. Surgical removal of the diseased pericardium may be necessary under these circumstances.

*Tuberculous pericarditis* occurs when the pericardium becomes infected by the tuberculosis bacterium. The pericardium may be involved alone or as part of a pulmonary or more generalized tuberculous infection. The pericardium becomes thick and densely scarred and the clinical manifestations may be similar to those of constrictive pericarditis. The treatment is the use of antituberculosis drugs. If the drugs fail to result in improvement, surgical removal of the pericardium may be necessary.

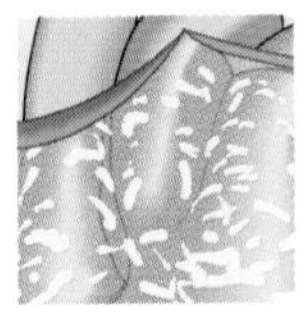

# The Pericardial Sac and Layers of the Heart Wall

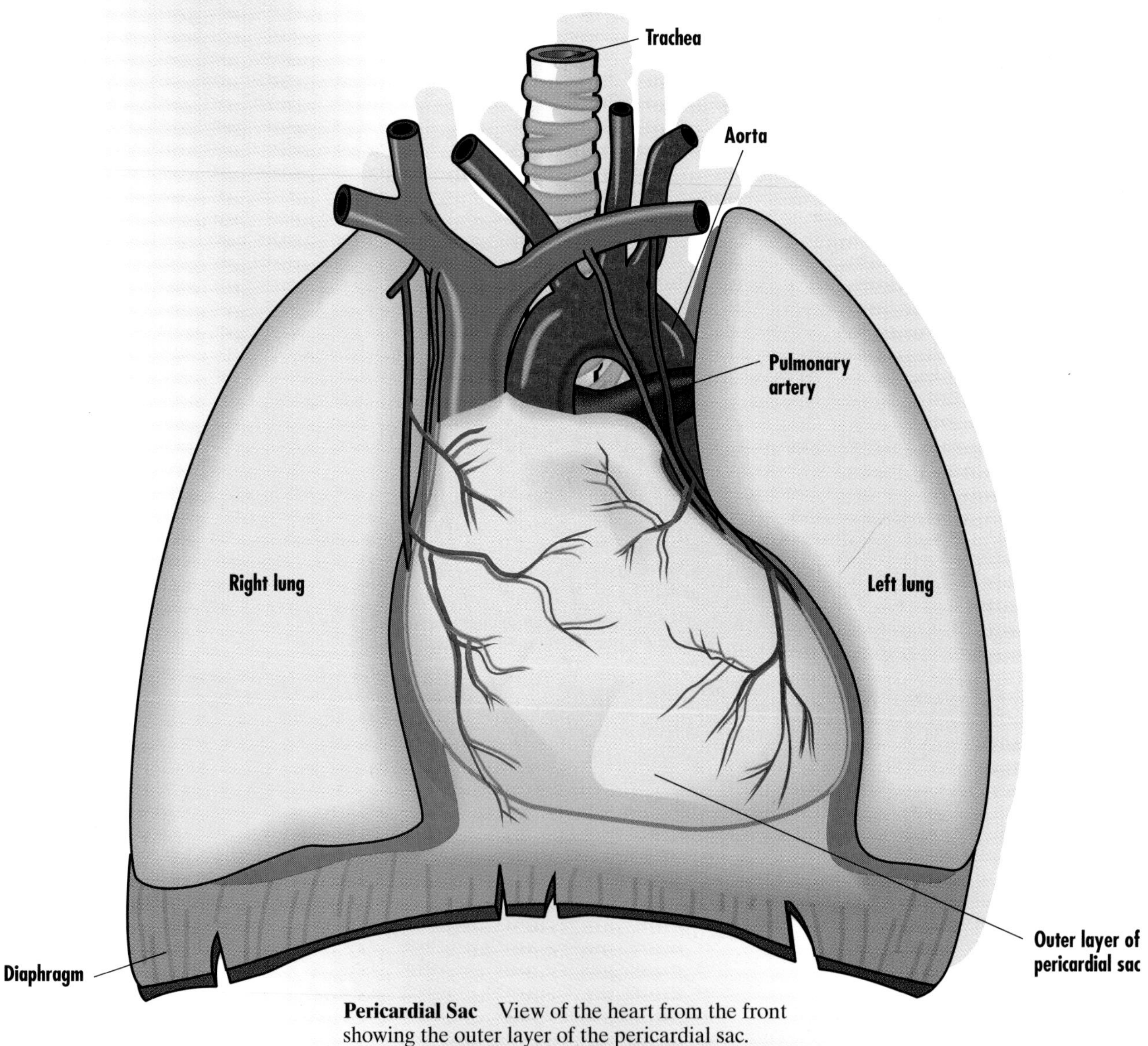


**Pericardial Sac** View of the heart from the front showing the outer layer of the pericardial sac.

**Layers of the Heart Wall** The thin outer layer is the *pericardium*; the thick middle layer is the muscular layer, the *myocardium*; and the inner lining of the heart is the *endocardium*.

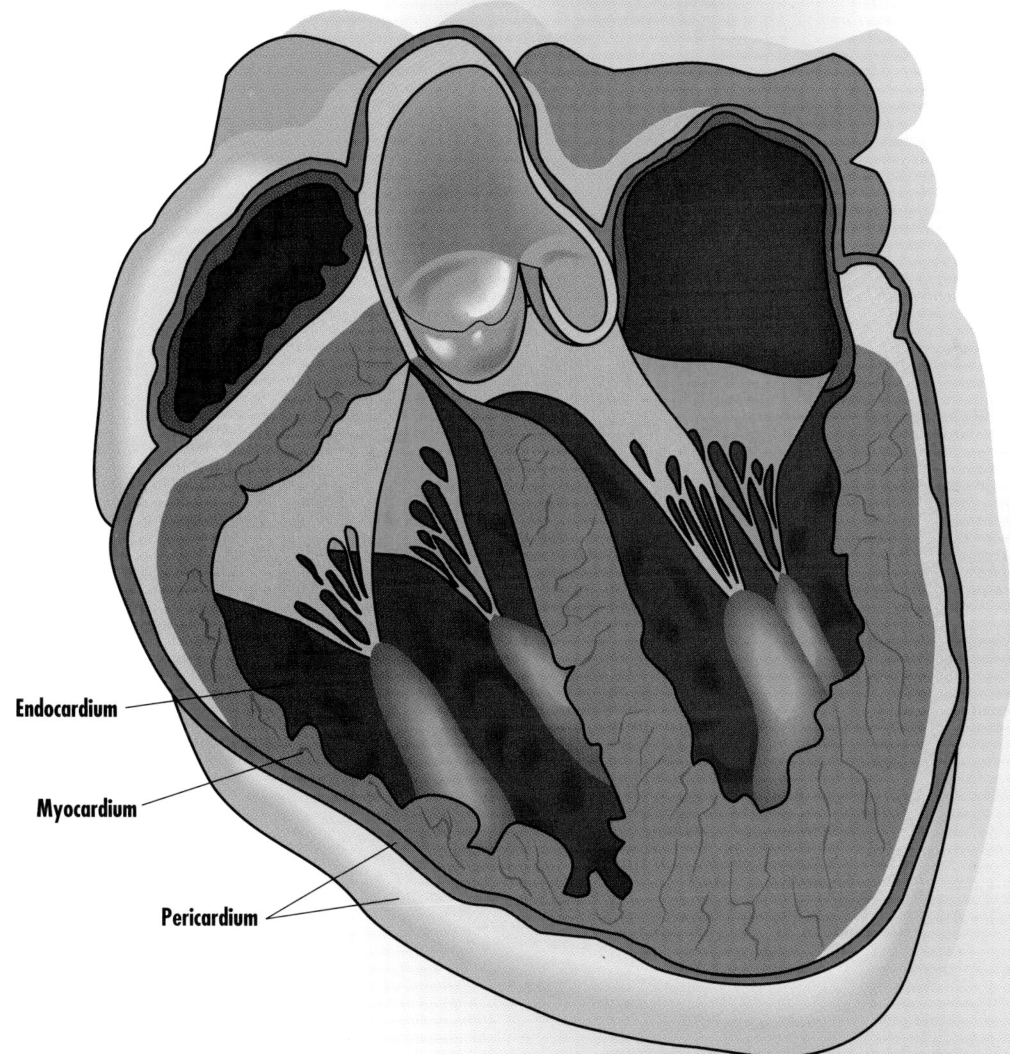

# Infections of the Heart

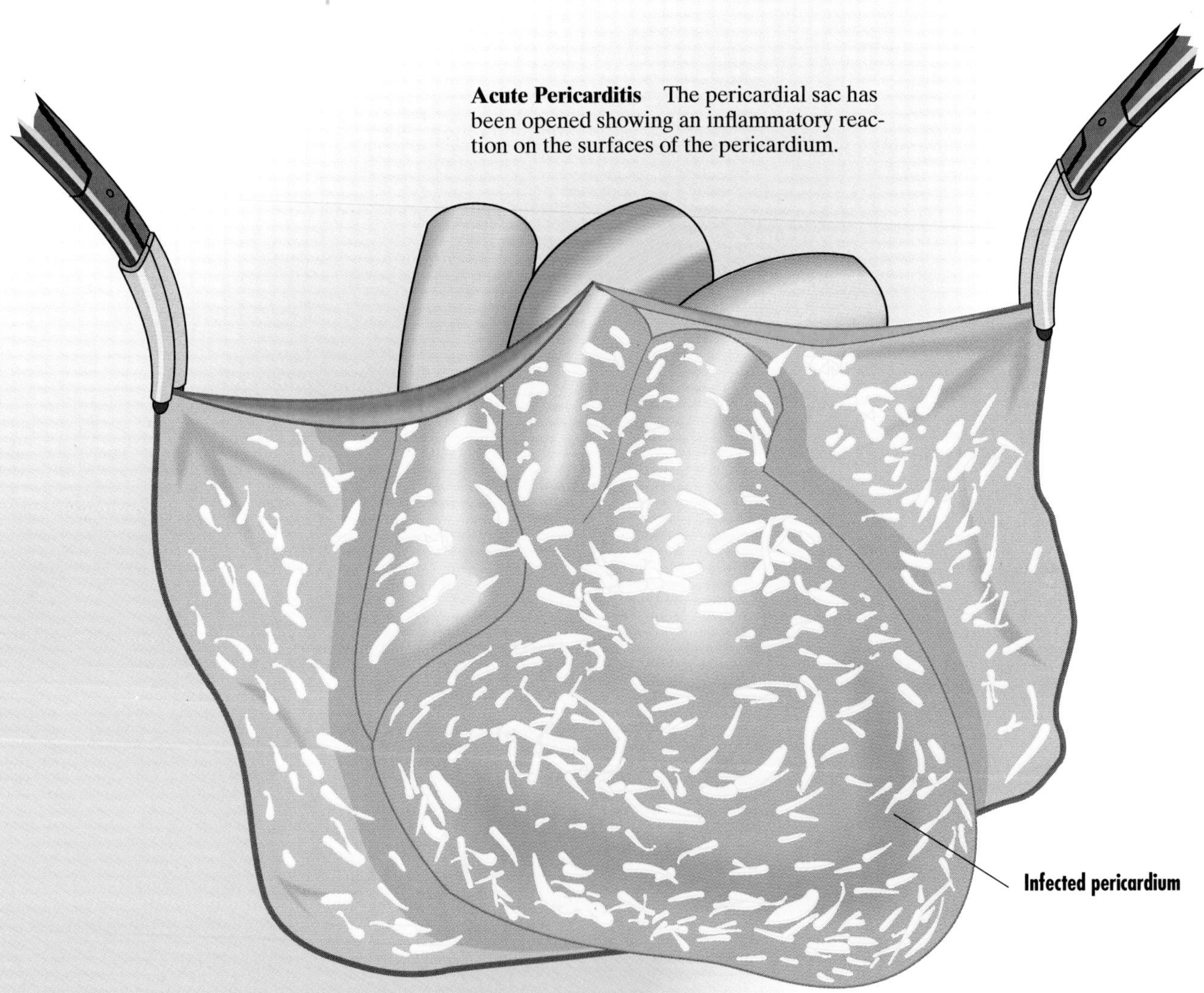


**Acute Pericarditis** The pericardial sac has been opened showing an inflammatory reaction on the surfaces of the pericardium.

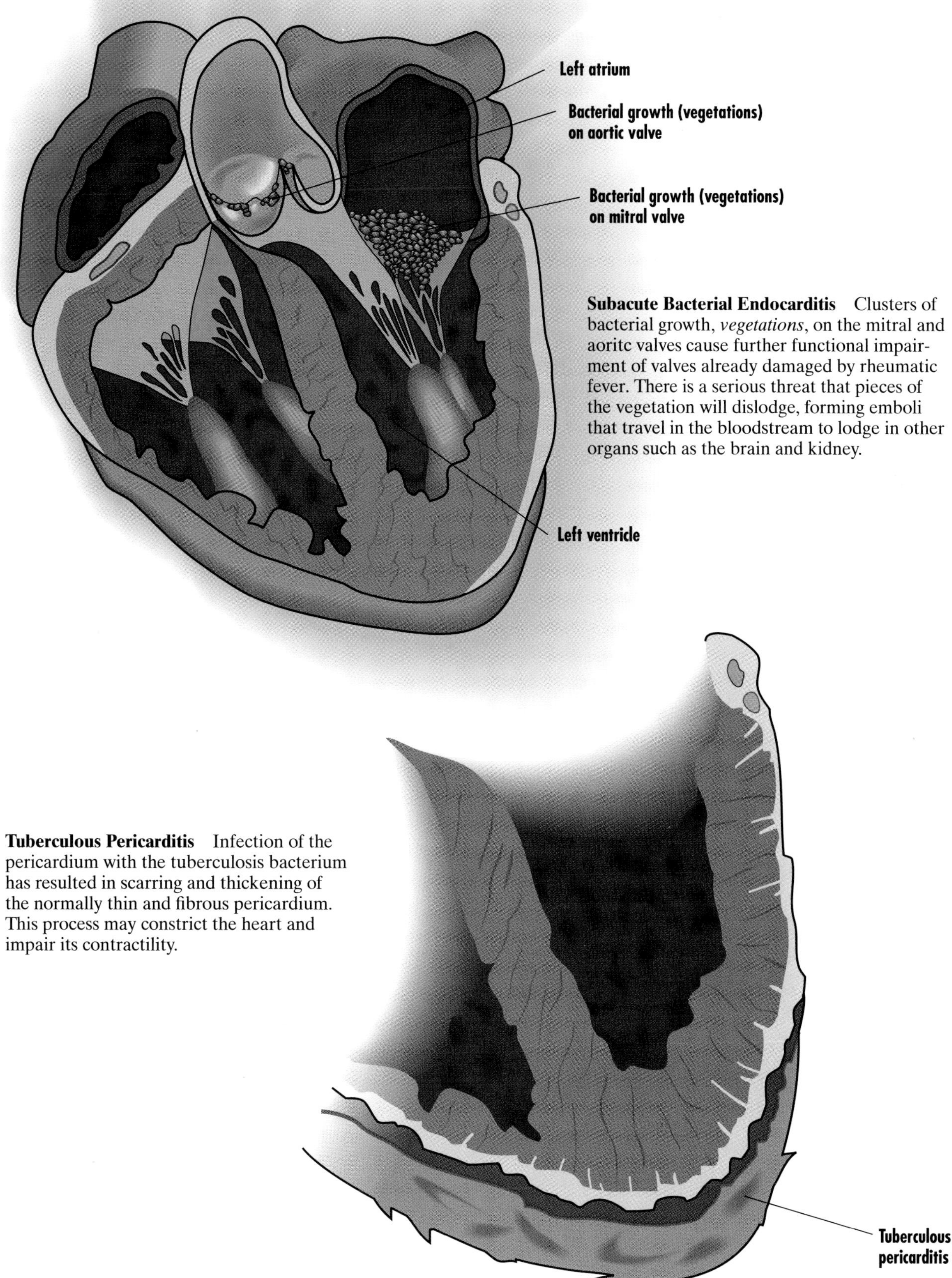


**Subacute Bacterial Endocarditis** Clusters of bacterial growth, *vegetations*, on the mitral and aoritc valves cause further functional impairment of valves already damaged by rheumatic fever. There is a serious threat that pieces of the vegetation will dislodge, forming emboli that travel in the bloodstream to lodge in other organs such as the brain and kidney.

**Tuberculous Pericarditis** Infection of the pericardium with the tuberculosis bacterium has resulted in scarring and thickening of the normally thin and fibrous pericardium. This process may constrict the heart and impair its contractility.

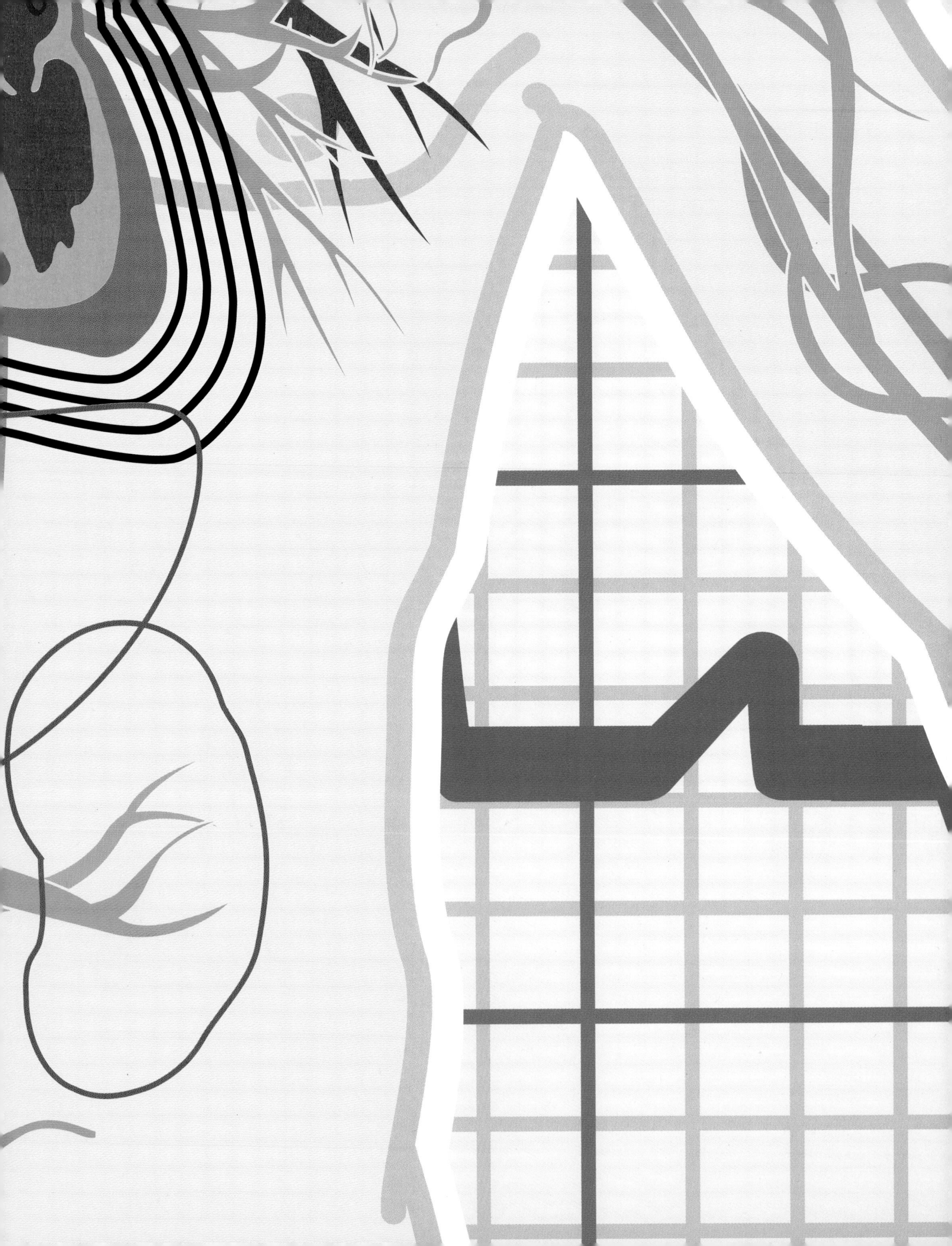

PART 5

# THE ABNORMAL VASCULAR SYSTEM

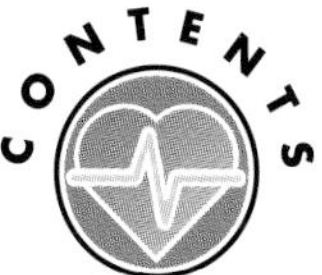

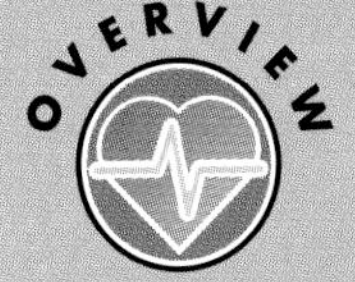
OVERVIEW

IN PARTS 1 THROUGH 4 of *How Your Heart Works,* we have concentrated on the heart, discussing its anatomy and physiology, the examination of the cardiac patient, and the major cardiac abnormalities. We turn now to the vascular component of the cardiovascular system and the role it plays in health and disease.

It was formerly thought that the vascular system played a passive role in the circulation of the blood, acting only as a delivery system of blood and oxygen that were supplied to it by the heart and lungs. We now recognize that the vascular system plays an active, dynamic role, working in close conjunction with the heart. In addition to its supportive role, the vascular system is responsible for many of the clinical manifestations of cardiovascular diseases.

In Part 5 we will address three particularly important cardiovascular problems in which the vascular system plays a major role—shock, hypertension, and diseases of the aorta and peripheral vascular system. We will discuss the different types of shock and note that their common denominator is actually a mechanism attributable to the vascular system.

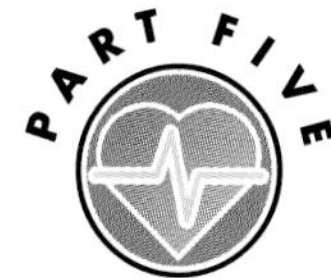


Although the heart is a major target organ of hypertension and bears a significant burden imposed by the disease, hypertension is not primarily a disease of the heart. As we shall see, many factors outside the heart play important roles in the production of hypertension. The vascular system, particularly the elastic and muscular components of the arterial wall, plays a significant role in the control of normal blood pressure and in the production of hypertension. We will also discuss the importance of the kidneys, nervous system, and endocrine glands in both normal and high blood pressure.

Finally, we will discuss certain specific disorders of the aorta and other blood vessels.

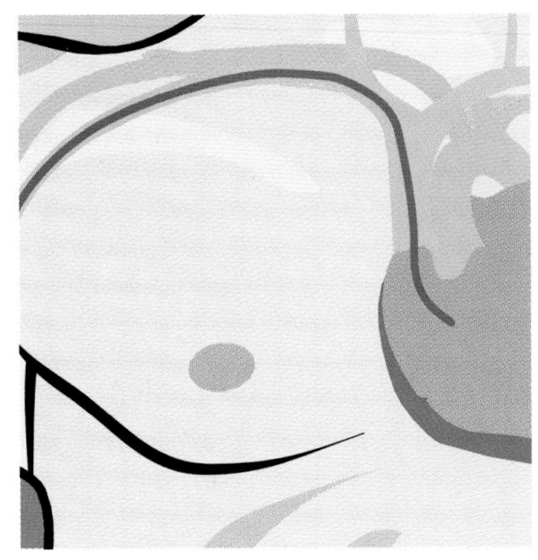

# Circulatory Shock

THE BODY MAY experience several types of circulatory shock. The common denominator of shock is a persistent deficiency of blood flow to the tissues, which usually occurs suddenly but may also be gradual and insidious. Inadequate perfusion of tissues with oxygenated blood leads to a progressive, eventually irreversible, deterioration of cellular and organ function, and ultimately to death. Extreme circulatory failure and shock can be caused by any one or a combination of three major mechanisms.

*Cardiogenic shock* is due to a critical reduction in cardiac filling or emptying, and the resultant rapid and severe decrease in cardiac output, despite adequate blood volume within the vascular system. Cardiogenic shock is encountered most commonly after an acute myocardial infarction, but may also occur as a result of aortic stenosis, mitral regurgitation, myocarditis, or severe arrhythmias, any of which impairs cardiac output. Loss of myocardial function after cardiac arrest or surgery may also precipitate shock. A severe restriction of cardiac filling, such as may occur due to an excessive amount of fluid in the pericardial sac, called *pericardial tamponade*, produces a similar effect. When caused by infarction, cardiogenic shock is generally associated with a 40% or more reduction of left ventricular myocardial function.

*Hypovolemic (low-volume) shock* results from any condition that critically reduces the blood volume. Blood volume may be reduced by loss of whole blood, such as occurs in a hemorrhage, or loss of plasma, the liquid component of blood, such as occurs in burns and infections. The most common causes of an acute and significant hemorrhage are severe trauma that tears a major blood vessel or damages an internal organ such as the spleen or liver, and bleeding from the gastrointestinal tract secondary to an ulcer or cirrhosis of the liver. Defects in blood-clotting mechanisms may contribute to bleeding and blood volume loss. The most common causes of decreases in plasma volume include severe burns, severe inflammations of the skin, and dehydration due to excessive vomiting, diarrhea, or an inadequate intake of fluids.

The severity of hypovolemic shock is related to the degree of blood volume loss and the rapidity with which the loss occurs. It is generally estimated that the sudden loss of 25% or more of an individual's vascular volume overwhelms compensatory mechanisms and produces shock.

The third mechanism for the production of shock occurs as a result of generalized vasodilation or *distributive shock* resulting from exposure to toxic substances produced by bacteria (*septic shock)*; allergic reactions to drugs, insect stings, or foods *(anaphylactic shock)*; overdoses of drugs that cause vasodilation; or severe trauma to the brain or spinal cord *(neurogenic shock)*. All of these types of shock produce an increase in blood vessel capacity without a corresponding increase in blood volume, resulting in a state of relative low blood volume and a decrease in cardiac output.

Although most cases of circulatory shock can be classified into one of these general types, many patients in shock have features of two or more, even all of these types.

The patient in shock may be unconscious, be in a stage of semiconsciousness or stupor, or be fully conscious. He or she appears alarmingly pallid, with skin discoloration that is often described as ashen gray. The skin is almost always cold and sweaty, often described as "clammy," although by contrast in distributive shock the skin may be warm (*warm shock)* because of enlarged blood vessels. The level of the arterial systolic blood pressure is below 80 to 90 millimeters of mercury in patients who previously had a normal blood pressure, but may be higher in patients who were previously hypertensive. In severe shock, the blood pressure may be too low to detect by the usual method.

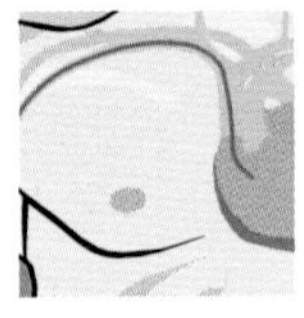

In response to the reduction in arterial blood pressure and tissue perfusion, the body initiates compensatory mechanisms in an effort to combat the circulatory shock. Pressure receptors (*baroreceptors)* within the carotid arteries and aorta are sensitive to the fall in blood pressure and respond with stimulation of the sympathetic nervous system, resulting in arterial and venous vasoconstriction, an increased heart rate, and increased contractility of the heart. These results are mediated by a variety of humoral and hormonal chemical substances that are secreted by the adrenal and pituitary glands and by the kidneys. They decrease the capacity of the vascular system and redistribute blood to guarantee brain, kidney, and heart perfusion at the expense of the skin, intestines, and skeletal muscle.

Another compensatory mechanism is increased absorption of fluid into the bloodstream from the tissues. This interstitial fluid is normally located outside the vascular system (extravascular) and cells (extacellular), but in the shock state it is absorbed into the blood vessels, thereby increasing the vascular volume.

As shock continues and progresses, there is increased cell injury and cell death. This is associated with the release of toxic substances into the blood that alter the critical acid-base and electrolyte balance of the blood, reinforcing the shock state, and that eventually result in "irreversible" shock. This is the terminal stage of shock where the body is unable to respond favorably to treatment and death results.

The prevention of circulatory shock is a prime objective in the treatment of a seriously ill patient, for whom the development of shock is a distinct possibility. Prompt and effective therapy of infections, careful handling of seriously injured patients, investigation into possible allergies and bleeding tendencies, and avoidance of agents that promote hemorrhage are examples of measures that must be included in prevention.

If the condition of preshock is recognized, measures to prevent progress to shock are vital. The management of the patient who is already in shock involves three general principles: determine the underlying cause of the shock, decide upon measures to remedy the cause, and provide cardiovascular support. Because of the urgency of the situation, all of these measures are performed simultaneously.

The patient in a state of shock is best managed in the intensive care unit (ICU) of a hospital where continuous monitoring of vital signs (pulse, respiration, blood pressure, body temperature), the electrocardiogram, and other factors such as central venous pressure, can be done. Monitoring the central venous pressure is a valuable index of the state of the circulation and fluid balance. Elevations of venous pressure indicate a severe threat of overloading the heart and the possibility of pump failure.

Urinary output is also a valuable measue to monitor in the patient in shock. An output of at least one ounce of urine per hour is considered adequate, but because of excessive reabsorption of tissue fluid by the patient in shock, this may fall to about two-thirds of an ounce per hour. The laboratory is valuable in helping the physician monitor important factors such as kidney function, acid-base balance, blood oxygen, and levels of electrolytes such as potassium, sodium, magnesium, and chloride. The physician, guided by the laboratory findings, is able to correct deficiencies and excesses if they occur.

Cardiogenic shock is most frequently due to an acute myocardial infarction, and cardiovascular support is essential. Unless cardiac output can be maintained, the patient will die. The mortality rate of patients in cardiogenic shock is 70% to 90%.

In the acute phase of a myocardial infarction, the systolic function of the heart can be improved by the administration of pharmacologic agents that mimic the action of the sympathetic nervous system to stimulate myocardial contractility, promote vasoconstriction, and increase the heart rate. These actions improve general circulation and, most importantly, the coronary circulation. Several agents are available that, if promptly administered intravenously, help in dissolving the clot component of the obstruction occluding the coronary artery.

A recent development has been the use of a balloon pump, which is inserted into the aorta and helps increase coronary blood flow by its pumping action. Studies have shown that the balloon pump is especially helpful in those patients who receive clot-dissolving agents.

Although still regarded as investigational therapy in acute myocardial infarction and cardiogenic shock, balloon dilation, or angioplasty, has been used to open the occluded coronary artery and thereby increase coronary circulation. Additionally, a number of patients have undergone open heart revascularizing surgery for the treatment of acute myocardial infarction with accompanying cardiogenic shock.

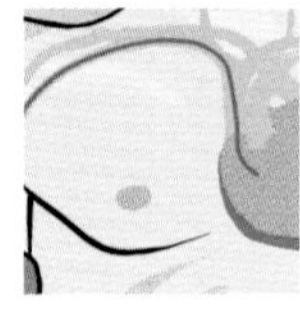

Both of these therapies require preliminary diagnostic coronary angiocardiography and qualify as aggressive therapy, especially in a patient who is already seriously ill. Although the available data indicate that, in many cases, restoration of the coronary circulation provides the best opportunity for survival, these procedures can only be done when proper facilities are available, and with the full support of the family and, if feasible, the patient. The decision to perform either of these procedures should be based on the physician's estimate of the probability of success coupled with the desires of the patient and family.

In cases of cardiac arrest due to cessation of heart action or the presence of a serious and ineffective cardiac rhythm such as ventricular fibrillation, cardiopulmonary resuscitation should be instituted immediately. Details of the technique will be presented later in this book. Under these circumstances, the use of electric shock by a defibrillator is often used in an attempt to restore effective heart action by restoration of independent cardiac action.

An artificial pacemaker may be used as a valuable adjunct in providing cardiovascular support to a patient in cardiogenic shock who has an ineffective cardiac rate or rhythm. The pacemaker provides a stimulus for myocardial contraction.

The use of artificial pacemakers is not confined to those patients in cardiogenic shock. They are used extensively in patients, usually elderly, with ischemic heart disease who have recurrent or continuous arrhythmias that jeopardize cardiac output.

Artificial pacemakers may be placed externally or internally in the chest wall. They must be monitored carefully to make sure that their power source, usually batteries, is adequate. There is an increasing use of atomic-powered artificial pacemakers.

In case of hypovolemic shock, increasing intravascular volume is essential. When volume depletion is due to massive hemorrhage, blood transfusions are the treatment of choice. Plasma is used in conditions where plasma loss has resulted in low vascular volume such as in burns or severe infections. Intravenous infusion of large amounts of fluid may be necessary to restore vascular volume. Saline (salt) solutions should be administered with caution since their use in the elderly and in those with known preexisting heart conditions may lead to abnormal retention of fluid and congestive heart failure.

In distributive shock, the main therapeutic effort is against the offending agent. Vigorous antibiotic therapy should be used in septic shock. Epinephrine (adrenalin) and corticosteroids (prednisone, for example) may be life-saving in the event of allergic reactions or anaphylactic shock. Vasoconstrictor drugs are useful in treating distributive shock due to overdoses of vasodilator drugs. The treatment of neurogenic shock depends on the underlying neurologic disorder.

# Circulatory Shock

**Characteristic Appearance of a Patient in Shock**
The patient is unconscious and the skin is pale and cold. The blood pressure is low, and the pulse is rapid and weak. An arrhythmia may be present. The status of the neck veins and the venous pressure are very helpful in evaluating the circulatory condition. In an intensive care unit, this patient would be constantly monitored by an electocardiogram and mechanical determination of the blood pressure. Urinary output would be monitored by a bladder catheter.

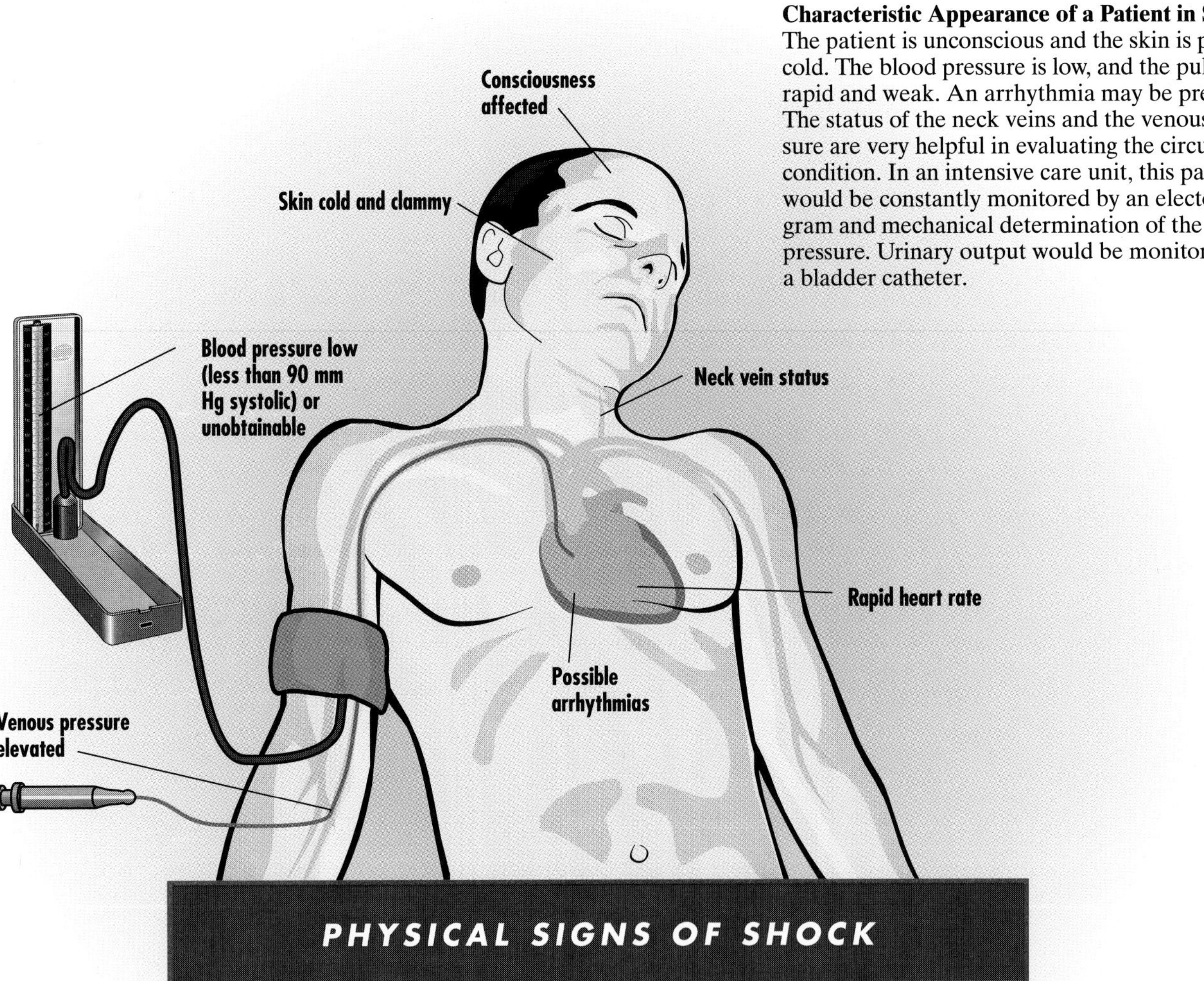


## PHYSICAL SIGNS OF SHOCK

**Conscious/Semiconscious/Unconscious**

**Abnormal Skin Pallor and Low Temperature**

**Rapid Heart Rate**

**Electrocardiogram**
Arrhythmias
Acute Myocardial Infarction

**Low Blood Pressure**

**Status of Venous Pressure**
Elevated: Fluid Overload
Low: Expansion of Volume Needed

**Status of Neck Veins**
Collapsed: Fluids Needed
Distended: Fluid Overload, Danger of Pump Failure

**Compensatory Mechanisms** When the body is in shock, it initiates mechanisms that attempt to compensate for the effects of circulatory shock. These compensatory processes produce the cold, clammy skin and the rapid heart rate so evident in the shock state. Three of these mechanisms are constriction of the arteries of muscle, skin, and abdominal organs to favor circulation of blood to the heart and brain; rapid heart rate; and increased kidney absorption of sodium and fluid.

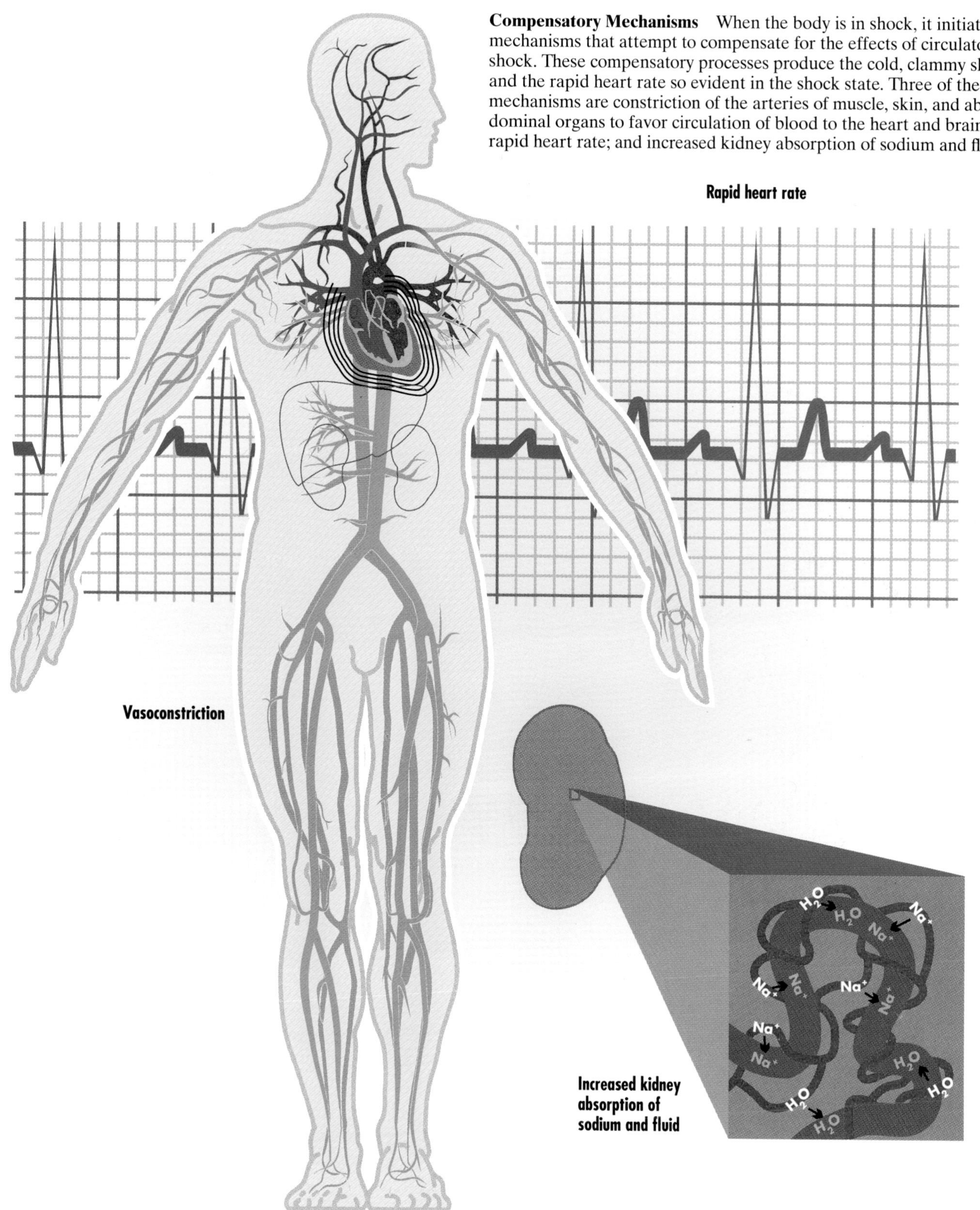

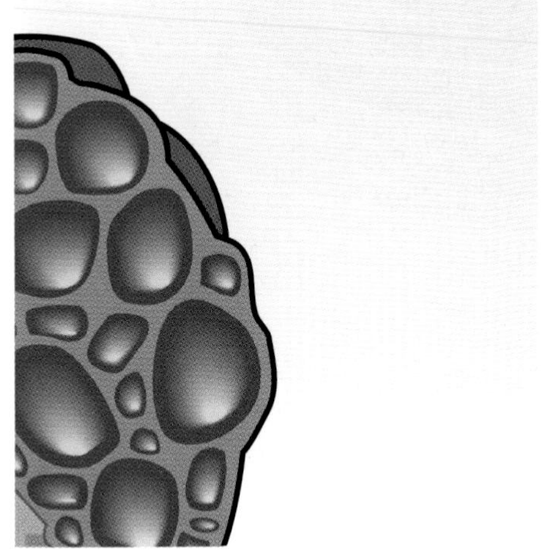

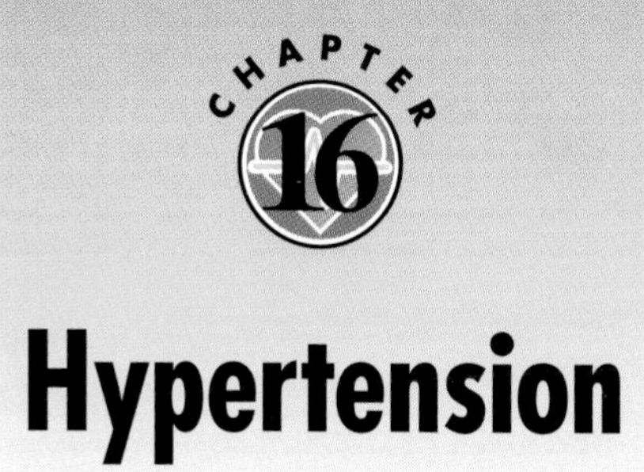

# Hypertension

HYPERTENSION IS A major health problem; more than 58 million persons in the United States have hypertension. Of all diseases, hypertension accounts for the largest number of outpatient prescriptions. It is especially common in the elderly population, with about two-thirds of this group over age 65 having elevated blood pressures.

Hypertension may be defined as a persistent elevation of the resting systolic blood pressure to 140 millimeters of mercury (mm Hg) or above, and/or an elevation of the diastolic pressure to 90 mm Hg or above. Hypertensive blood pressure levels in children are substantially lower. Several subgroups of hypertension have been defined.

For several years before persistent elevated blood pressure develops in the patient, transient rises in pressure to abnormal levels may occur during stressful situations; this condition is called *labile hypertension*. Some, but not all, of these individuals later develop chronic hypertension. The stronger the family history of hypertension, the more likely is the person with transient elevations of blood pressure to develop persistent hypertension.

In many older individuals, the systolic pressure alone is elevated, which is known as *isolated systolic hypertension*. This condition is usually an adjustment to increased resistance in the arterial system due to arteriosclerosis and usually is not a cause for clinical concern.

*Accelerated* or *malignant hypertension* is defined by sustained or sudden diastolic blood pressure higher than 125 mm Hg plus evidence of damage to the heart, brain, kidneys, or eyes, which are the major organ systems affected by hypertension. The term malignant hypertension is reserved for patients in whom examination of the retina shows swelling or "choking" of the optic nerve disc. This situation requires hospitalization and an urgent diagnostic workup and treatment, since the course is usually rapidly downhill and fatal.

There are many causes of hypertension, but 90% of patients are in the category of *essential hypertension*, the causes of which have not as yet been defined. The remaining 10% of patients have *secondary hypertension*, which means it is associated with and due to an underlying disease. These secondary types of hypertension are important to recognize because many conditions are amenable to corrective surgery.

Although the cause of essential hypertension is unknown, intensive research has resulted in an understanding of several mechanisms that contribute to its development. Patients with essential hypertension do not have a uniform profile, and there is evidence that multiple factors, varying from patient to patient, may operate either alone or in combination with other factors to cause the disease. Studies of families indicate that 20% to 40% of cases of essential hypertension have a genetic basis; recent research has identified abnormalities in gene structure that may play a role in its development.

The one characteristic that patients with essential hypertension have in common is increased resistance in the vascular system. It is this increased resistance that requires increased blood pressure to effectively maintain adequate organ and tissue perfusion with blood and oxygen. Several organ systems play roles in the development of the increased vascular resistance.

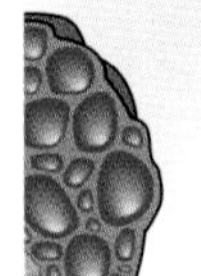

Attention has been focused on the role of the kidneys in the development of essential hypertension. Studies of the kidneys of hypertensive patients have shown defective handling of sodium, a component of sodium chloride or ordinary salt. The kidneys tend to absorb an excessive amount of sodium from tissue fluid. Sodium attracts fluid, resulting in an expansion of the circulatory volume and increased resistance to the pumping action of the heart. It has been shown that populations with diets low in sodium usually have fewer people with hypertension. Similarly, hypertension can be produced in animals by the administration of a diet with a high sodium content.

There is evidence that the sympathetic nervous system of the hypertensive patient overreacts to stimuli such as emotional stress, cold, and exercise. This means an increased production of, and an exaggerated response to, certain substances that cause vasoconstriction, an increased heart rate, and other changes that result in an increase in blood pressure. This overactivity of the sympathetic nervous system has been noted in the children of some hypertensive patients and indicates the likely future development of hypertension in the children.

The role of the *renin-angiotensin system* in the development of essential hypertension has also been the subject of intense investigation. Renin is an enzyme produced by the kidney that converts a protein produced by the liver into a substance known as angiotensin I. Angiotensin I is, in turn, converted into angiotensin II by an enzyme in the plasma called angiotensinogen. Angiotensin II is a potent vasoconstrictor and a stimulant for the excretion of a powerful adrenal gland hormone called aldosterone, which is responsible for the retention of water and salt. This cascade of events is thought to play an important role in some patients with hypertension. The genes regulating the production of renin and angiotensinogen have been identified and research is underway on the abnormal forms of these genes that may account for problems with the renin-angiotensin system.

The kidneys are also responsible for the production of substances referred to as kinins that cause vasodilation. In the absence of these substances, vasodilation and renal excretion of sodium both may be impaired, which also would produce an increased vascular resistance.

Finally, *obesity* is an important contributing factor of the development of hypertension, although the mechanism of its action is unknown.

Although secondary hypertension accounts for 10% or fewer cases of hypertension, it is important to recognize, since many of the causes are correctable. Included here are some of the underlying diseases causing secondary hypertension: insufficient blood supply to one or both kidneys; certain tumors of the kidneys, parathyroid glands, and brain; diseases or tumors of the adrenal glands that cause an excessive production of substances that affect blood pressure; coarctation of the aorta—a constricting lesion of the aorta that causes increased resistance to the pumping action of the heart; infections or other diseases of the kidney that reduce kidney function; certain medications, such as oral contraceptives, in some patients; lead poisoning; and neurologic disorders.

Another cause of hypertension is pregnancy. Pregnancy-induced hypertension, formerly called preeclampsia, involves widespread vasoconstriction. It tends to occur during the first pregnancy, particularly in mothers under the age of 20, in twin pregnancies, or in diabetic patients. It must be differentiated from preexisting essential or secondary hypertension that has been aggravated by the pregnancy. The condition accelerates toward the end of pregnancy and is often associated with edema and the presence of albumin (a protein) in the urine. During pregnancy, treatment of hypertension requires special therapy and precautions. In patients with pregnancy-induced hypertension, blood pressure returns to normal shortly after delivery.

Secondary hypertension should be considered in patients under the age of 40, in patients with severe hypertension, and in patients whose hypertension is difficult to control. The history and physical examination will often provide the physician with clues that will lead to the suspicion of secondary hypertension. The physician then has available a wide variety of laboratory and other diagnostic aids that will establish the diagnosis of the underlying disease and lead to appropriate corrective therapy. However, these studies are costly and some are potentially risky. Thus, if the blood pressure elevation is mild or moderate and responsive to therapy, only a minimal diagnostic workup is considered necessary. In patients with accelerated or malignant hypertension, intensive studies are always warranted after pressure is lowered and stabilized to detect any potentially correctable cause of the hypertension.

Most patients with hypertension have no symptoms. The diagnosis is usually made under two circumstances: first, by detection of an elevated blood pressure during a physical examination for health insurance or for some unrelated condition; or second, by the development of a complication from the hypertension that requires medical attention. Hypertension itself is not a problem, but the damage it does to certain organs can be extremely serious.

Cardiac complications are the most commonly seen effects of hypertension. They include congestive heart failure, coronary heart disease manifested as angina pectoris or acute myocardial infarction, and disorders of the aorta and peripheral vascular system. The central nervous system manifestations of hypertension include headache, dizziness, and the more serious complication of stroke—cerebral thrombosis or hemorrhage. Kidney failure may develop from hypertension. Eye manifestations include changes in visual acuity and blurring of vision. Eye changes may be the first manifestations of malignant hypertension.

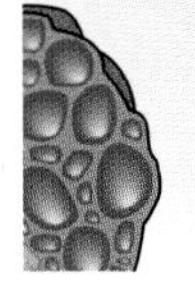

For a patient with essential hypertension, a thorough history and physical examination, including the ophthalmoscopic examination of the retina, are essential. The electrocardiogram offers a valuable assessment of the cardiac damage that may have occurred. The general laboratory is helpful in evaluating kidney function and in identifying additional risk factors such as diabetes and high levels of blood cholesterol.

The goals of antihypertensive therapy are to lower blood pressure and to prevent complications. Complications that are already present should be treated appropriately. Advances in pharmacologic technology have dramatically reduced the incidence of hypertensive complications such as congestive heart failure, kidney failure, stroke, and eye problems.

It is important to recognize the significance of the nonpharmacologic treatment of hypertension. For mild or moderate uncomplicated cases of hypertension, a trial of nonpharmacologic therapy should be tried and will often be successful. Measures would include a reduction in body weight if advisable, a reduction in dietary sodium intake, elimination of oral contraceptives and other possible hypertension-producing medications, initiation of an aerobic or dynamic exercise program, reduction of alcohol intake to less than 2 ounces a day, cessation of smoking, and treatment of concomitant medical conditions. Changes in lifestyle to avoid emotional and physical stress are recommended.

During the period of nonpharmacologic treatment, blood pressure should be monitored carefully because hypertension can increase in severity without specific antihypertensive therapy.

In patients with moderate to severe hypertension or in those with mild hypertension who have failed to respond to nonpharmacologic therapy, pharmacologic therapy is justified. Unless the situation is urgent, such as in malignant hypertension complicated by end-organ damage, most physicians use the step-care program first proposed by the Joint National Commission on High Blood Pressure in 1980. It is important to maintain the nonpharmacologic program in conjunction with the pharmacologic program.

The step-care program uses the principle of initially introducing a single drug, the choice of which is left to the physician's judgment. Depending on the patient's response, the first step of using a simple medication may be adequate to control the blood pressure; if not, a second drug should be added. If necessary, a third drug is added. It is recommended that only one drug of a specific category be used at a time, but switching to an alternate drug in the same category may be advisable if response is inadequate or side effects occur.

Several categories of antihypertensive pharmacologic drugs are available, each of which attacks a specific mechanism that contributes to hypertension and that may be significant in that specific patient. *Diuretics* are useful in promoting increased secretion of sodium and fluid. A variety of agents are available that block or inhibit the sympathetic nervous system. These include the beta blockers, such as propranolol, as well as other agents that act both on the brain and peripheral nervous system to inhibit sympathetic nervous system activity. *Vasodilators* such as hydralazine and minoxidil lower vascular resistance by their dilating action on blood vessels. Recently *ACE (angiotensin-converting enzyme) inhibitors* have been introduced. These medications block the enzymatic action of the enzyme angiotensinogen, thus preventing conversion of angiotensin I to the potent vasoconstrictor angiotensin II. The *calcium channel blockers* are agents that have a variety of cardiovascular actions. Most of the calcium blockers are effective in the treatment of essential hypertension because of their vasodilatory activity.

Once effective hypertensive control is accomplished, a step-down program should be initiated by the physician. This involves a gradual decrease in the dosage of drugs being used in the program, as well as discontinuing, on a trial basis, one drug at a time. Blood pressure should be carefully monitored during the step-down program.

Most patients with hypertension have no symptoms even though the target organs may be suffering permanent damage. For this reason, hypertension is often referred to as the "silent killer." Most patients are unaware of the potential dangers of untreated hypertension. More than 90% of essential hypertension can be controlled by one, two, or three pharmacologic agents. Following a drug regimen carefully is extremely important. To aid in patient compliance, most medications can be administered once or twice a day. The physician should be constantly on the alert for the occurrence of adverse reactions to the antihypertensive drugs as well as to interactions between them and other medications.

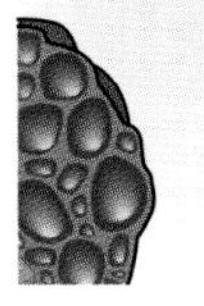

# When Is Your Blood Pressure Too High?

Hypertension that is untreated can lead to damage to a number of organs, including the heart, kidneys, eyes, and central nervous system. Heart problems are the most common, and changes in the eye are often the first sign of hypertension.

**Hypertensive Blood Pressures in Children**

*Note: All measurements are in millimeters of mercury (mm Hg)*

|  | | |
|---|---|---|
| **Newborns** | | |
| | Less than 7 days (systolic) | 96 – 106 |
| | 8 - 30 days (systolic) | 104 – 110 |
| **Infants (up to 2 years)** | | |
| | Systolic | 112 – 118 |
| | Diastolic | 74 – 82 |
| **Children 3 – 5 years** | | |
| | Systolic | 116 – 124 |
| | Diastolic | 76 – 84 |
| **Children 6 – 9 years** | | |
| | Systolic | 122 – 130 |
| | Diastolic | 78 – 86 |
| **Children 10 – 12 years** | | |
| | Systolic | 126 – 134 |
| | Diastolic | 82 – 90 |
| **Children 13 – 15 years** | | |
| | Systolic | 136 – 144 |
| | Diastolic | 86 – 92 |
| **Adolescents (16 – 18 years)** | | |
| | Systolic | 142 – 150 |
| | Diastolic | 92 – 98 |

**Classification of Blood Pressure in Adults 18 Years of Age or Older**

| Diastolic Blood Pressure Range | Category |
|---|---|
| less than 85 | Normal |
| 85 – 89 | High normal |
| 90 – 104 | Mild hypertension |
| 105 – 114 | Moderate hypertension |
| above 115 | Severe hypertension |

# Some Effects of Untreated Hypertension

Hypertension can cause enlargement (hypertrophy) of the left ventricle, as shown in this heart. Such a problem is very likely to result in heart failure.

The retina on the left shows normal blood vessels and optic nerve. The retina on the right shows the effects of hypertension: hemorrhages, leakage of fluid (exudates), and blurring of the margins of the optic nerve disc ("choked disc"). This patient undoubtedly has blurred vision.

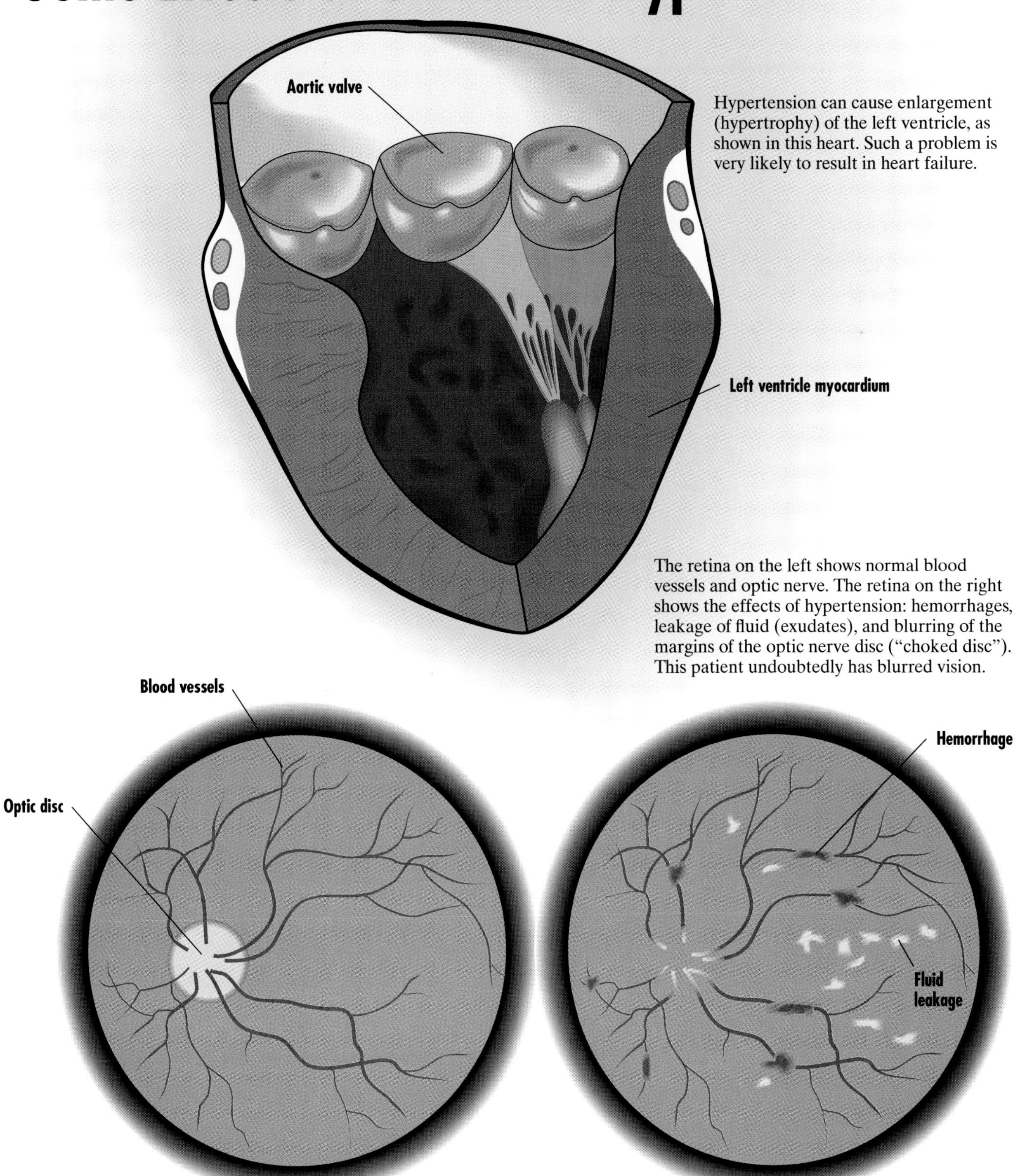

# How Hypertension Is Treated

All hypertension should be treated, but not all treatment involves medication. Changes in diet, regular exercise, and changes in lifestyle will often correct hypertension. If medication is necessary, several categories of drugs are available. Drug treatment is usually administered according to guidelines known as "step-care," which were developed by the Joint National Committee on Detection, Evaluation, and Treatment of High Blood Pressure.

## Step-Care Treatment of Hypertension

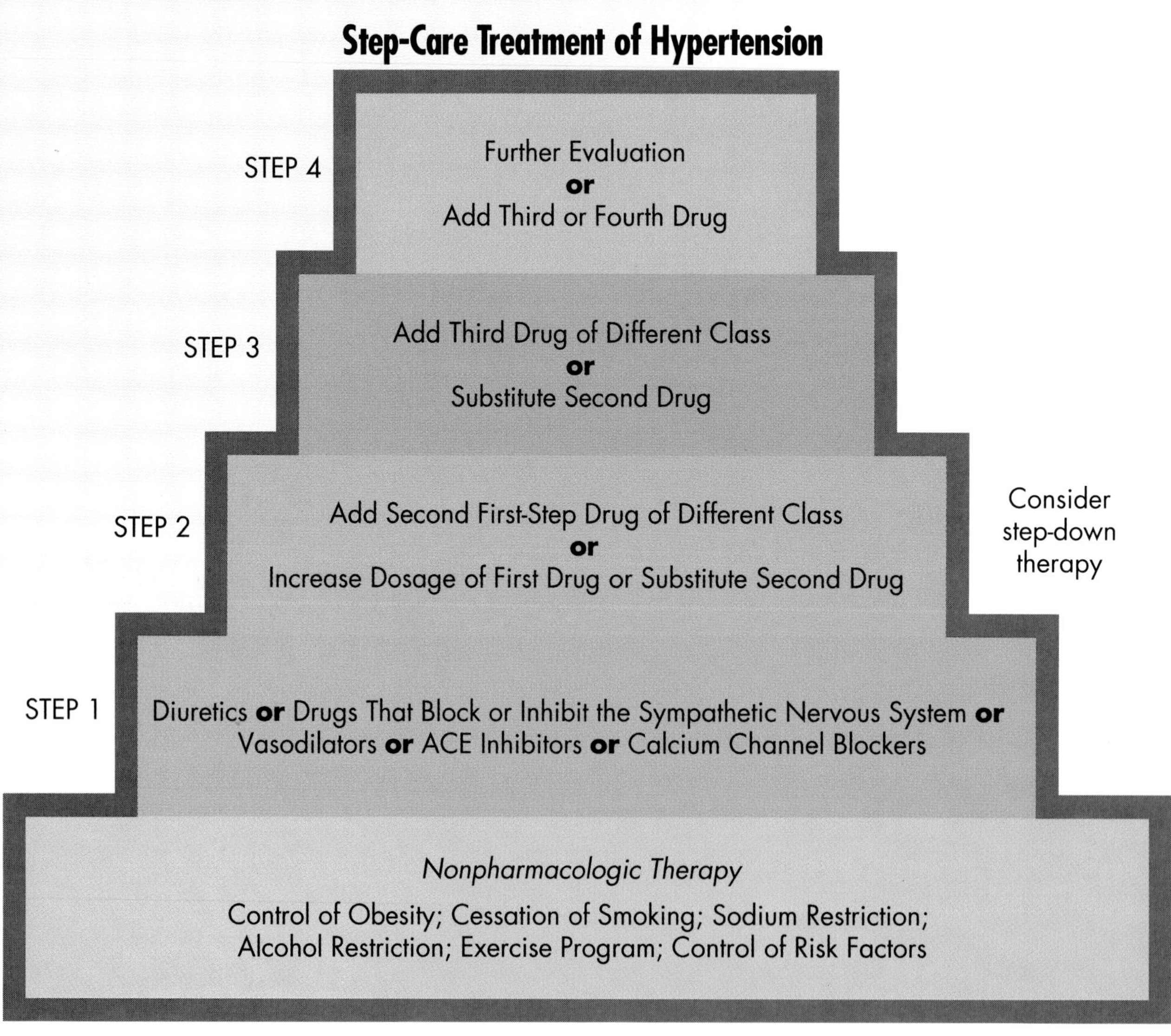


Adapted from the 1988 Report of the Joint National Committee on Detection, Evaluation, and Treatment of High Blood Pressure, by Sam Huntington.

# What Causes Secondary Hypertension?

Secondary hypertension can be caused by many factors. Three common causes—a restriction of the aorta (referred to as coarctation of the aorta, a congenital disease), kidney disorders, and adrenal gland tumors—are illustrated below.

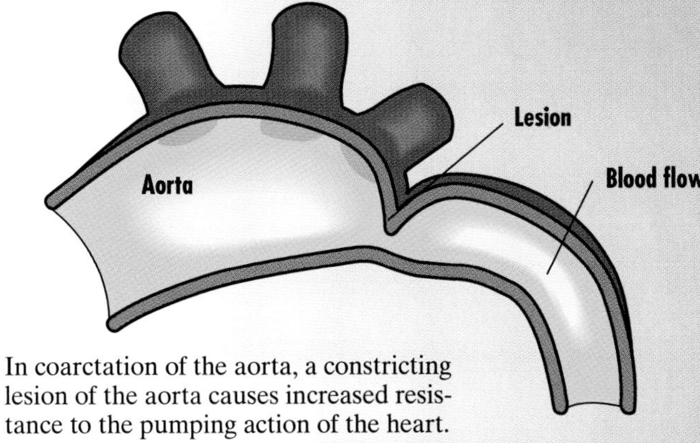


In coarctation of the aorta, a constricting lesion of the aorta causes increased resistance to the pumping action of the heart.

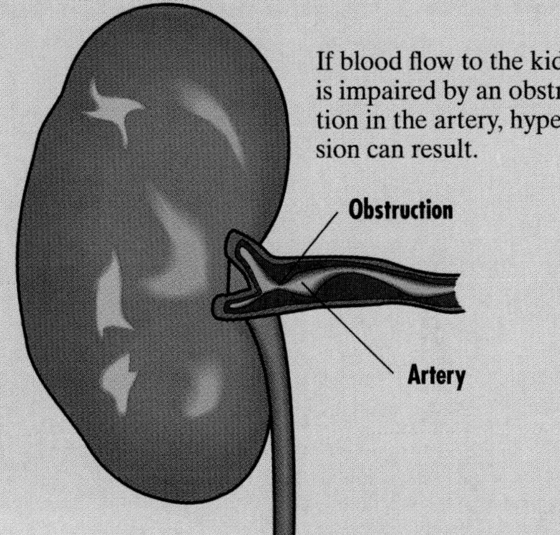


If blood flow to the kidney is impaired by an obstruction in the artery, hypertension can result.

Diseases of the kidney can reduce kidney function, resulting in hypertension. The lower part of the kidney illustrates the effect of a chronic kidney infection. The upper part of the kidney is an example of polycystic kidney disease, in which the numerous cysts impair kidney function.

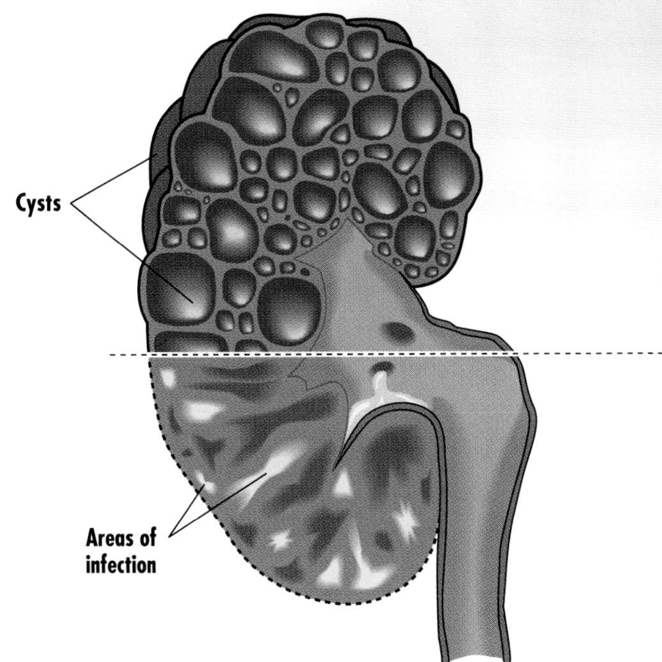


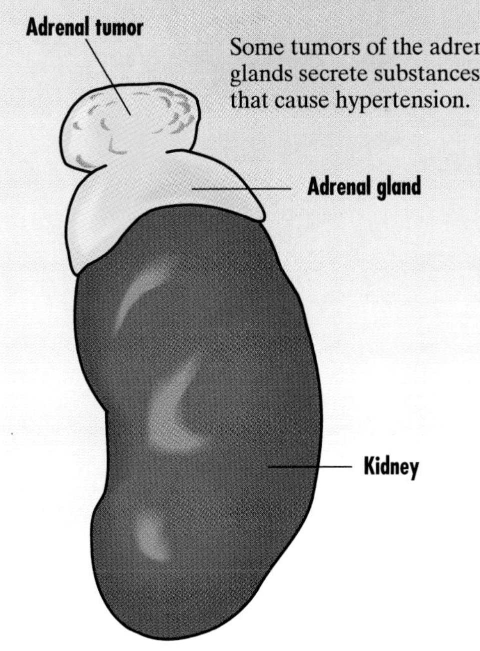


Some tumors of the adrenal glands secrete substances that cause hypertension.

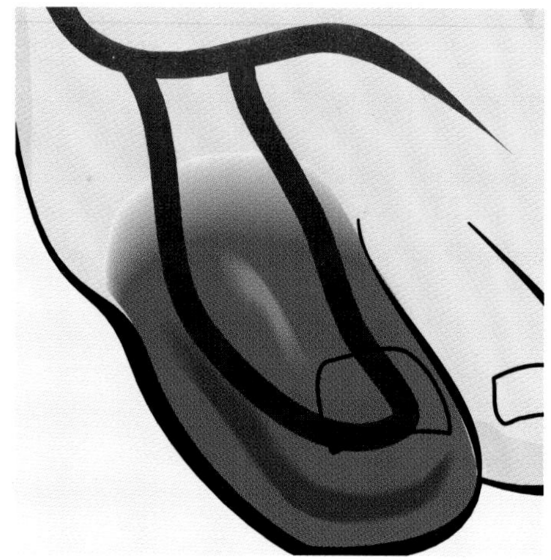

# Diseases of the Aorta and Peripheral Vascular System

THE AORTA AND the peripheral blood vessels share some of the diseases that we have previously considered when discussing the coronary artery circulation and coronary heart disease. Both the aorta and the peripheral arterial system are especially vulnerable to the development of atheromas and arteriosclerosis. In the case of the aorta, this may be related to the high pressure conveyed by each contraction of the left ventricle.

A chronic obstruction due to atherosclerosis occurring in the aorta usually involves the abdominal aorta and frequently extends past its point of division into the two large iliac arteries that supply blood to the lower extremities. The development of the obstruction is usually slow in progression, and the patient will often complain of pain in the hips and thighs occurring chiefly on exertion. The pain is referred to as *intermittent claudication*, and is caused by an inadequate supply of blood and oxygen to the tissues. Impotence is a common complaint in males because occlusion causes inadequacy of blood supply to the pelvic organs. The entire set of symptoms of aortoiliac obstruction is called Leriche's syndrome. Pallor, decreased skin temperature, and hair loss of the lower extremities may be present along with loss of pulses in the groin. The diagnosis is usually apparent by physical examination, measurement of pressure in the legs, and ultrasound analysis, but visualization of the aorta with radiopaque dye, a procedure called aortography, may be necessary. Surgical techniques are available to alleviate the obstruction. If the occlusion becomes complete or occurs suddenly because of a superimposed clot (thrombus), the deprivation of blood is a threat and may result in *gangrene,* or death of the tissues. Emergency surgery is needed and amputation may be necessary.

Atherosclerosis of the aorta is the most common cause of an aortic aneurysm, a balloon-like swelling of the aorta that is caused by weakening of the aortic wall. It may be a sacular outpouching or elongated (fusiform) dilation. Aneurysms may develop in any artery but are most commonly encountered in the aorta and brain. If not caused by atherosclerosis, an aneurysm is most likely congenital in origin.

Any portion of the aorta may be involved, but the abdominal aorta is the most common area involved. The aneurysm may produce no symptoms and is often detected on a physical examination done for some other reason. If the enlargement of the aneurysm progresses back toward the spine, abdominal and back pain may result. The diagnosis of an abdominal aneurysm is generally confirmed by ultrasound analysis or by computerized axial tomography (CAT) scan or by magnetic resonance imaging (MRI). Because of the concern about rupture, most physicians concur in the recommendation of surgical treatment if there is evidence that the aneurysm is enlarging. Various surgical techniques are available to repair or replace the aneurysm. Rupture of an abdominal aneurysm is a catastrophic event and often fatal because of the massive loss of blood that occurs. Emergency surgery may be effective in repairing the aorta after rupture.

An aneurysm of the upper or thoracic aorta that is close to its exit from the heart may be caused by several conditions other than atherosclerosis. It may be a late manifestation of syphilis. The spirochetal organism that causes syphilis may lodge in the tissues of the aorta and weaken the aortic wall. This condition is called syphilitic aortitis. Although syphilitic aneurysms rarely rupture, they may result in stretching of the aortic valve, which allows the development of severe aortic regurgitation. Syphilitic aneurysms of the aorta may grow very large and encroach on adjacent structures such as the esophagus, ribs, and spine. In addition, syphilitic aortitis may encroach on the orifices of some of the large branches of the aortic arch and cause vascular insufficiency of the organs they supply with blood.

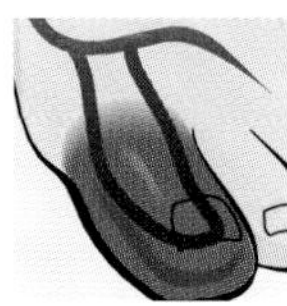

Another serious complication of aortic atherosclerosis is the development of a *dissecting aneurysm of the aorta.* A dissecting aneurysm results from the development of a tear in the inner lining or *intima* of the aorta as a result of damage to the intima by the atherosclerotic process. Hypertension is present in 80% to 90% of patients. The contractile power of the heart forces blood into the tear, and the blood then continues down the aorta between its layers, forming a fake channel or "double-barreled" aorta. The dissection may rupture back into the normal aortic channel and become a healed dissection, or it may rupture externally into the abdominal cavity with catastrophic loss of blood. The patient with aortic dissection experiences the sudden onset of severe pain that is sometimes difficult to distinguish from the pain of an acute myocardial infarction. The blood pressure is usually normal or elevated in an aortic dissection, whereas it drops following an infarction; this may give the physician a valuable clue concerning the diagnosis. The immediate treatment involves close monitoring, lowering the blood pressure, and reducing cardiac contractility. Emergency surgery, although sometimes necessary, has less likelihood of success than surgery following stabilization of the patient's condition.

In the peripheral arterial system, arteriosclerosis may lead to serious impairment of the circulation, especially of the lower extremities. This is a very common problem among smokers and a frequent complication of diabetes. As a result of an inadequate supply of blood and oxygen to the tissues of the legs, the patient may experience the muscle pain and fatigue of intermittent claudication. As narrowed arteries are unable to meet increased demands for oxygen, symptoms occur during exercise and are relieved by rest. If the arterial circulation becomes inadequate to satisfy the normal resting needs for oxygen, the sensation of cold or numbness occurs, and eventually gangrene may occur. The pulses in the feet may be decreased or absent. At this stage of the disease, every effort must be made to protect the feet against trauma and cold. Smoking has been demonstrated to have a serious adverse effect on the peripheral circulation and must be eliminated. The use of vasodilator drugs is of help in some patients, but in many cases the arteries are so diseased that they are incapable of dilating. Troublesome ulcers of the skin may develop that are generally resistant to treatment. Without treatment, gangrene may develop and amputation becomes necessary. Recent advances in graft surgery have resulted in successful replacement or bypass of diseased arteries with homografts or synthetic prostheses.

*Buerger's disease,* or *thromboangiitis obliterans,* is an uncommon disease that usually occurs in men between the ages of 20 and 40. The cause is unknown, but there is a definite relationship to smoking. Buerger's disease is characterized by an inflammatory reaction of the arteries, most commonly those of the lower extremities. The result is a gradual narrowing of the arteries, leading to insufficiency of blood and oxygen to the leg, and causing the patients to have pain in the leg muscles, usually after exertion. Treatment is difficult and usually unsatisfactory. Cessation of smoking is essential. Antibiotics may be useful, and there is limited value to the use of drugs that cause vasodilation. Tissue death may eventually result, leading to amputation.

*Raynaud's phenomenon* is characterized by periodic episodes of deficient blood supply to fingers or toes caused by vasoconstriction, apparently secondary to overactivity of the sympathetic nervous system. The disorder occurs most frequently in young women and may be a precursor of a generalized disease. Patients are extremely sensitive to the cold. Raynaud's phenomenon occurs chiefly in the upper extremities. The skin of the fingers becomes thin and pale as a result of deficient circulation. Slight trauma may lead to ulcerations, and, if the process continues, gangrenous changes may occur. If no underlying generalized disease is discovered, the disorder is referred to as Raynaud's disease. Treatment involves avoidance of cold and trauma. Treatment with medications that cause vasodilation by blocking the sympathetic nervous system may be helpful. In some cases, surgical removal of the sympathetic nervous supply to the arms has provided relief.

*Thrombophlebitis* is a common condition of the peripheral veins, especially those of the lower extremities. There is a tendency for clots (thrombi) to develop in the veins of the lower extremities if venous return is impaired. This may occur from prolonged bed rest because of illness or surgery, or from maintaining the legs in a dependent position for a prolonged period. Increased pressure within the abdomen that results from obesity or pregnancy also predisposes a person to the development of thrombi in the legs. In many cases, venous thrombi do not cause symptoms, but if they become infected, pain, tenderness, and redness of the skin will be present over the site of the involved vein. The veins involved may be deep in the tissues of the legs or superficial and close to the skin.

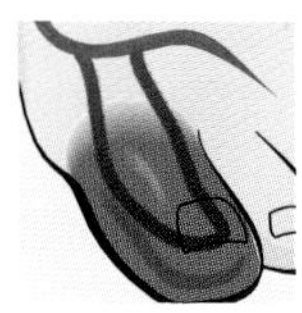

The danger of thrombophlebitis lies in the possibility of fragments of the thrombus dislodging and traveling through the blood as emboli. The emboli reach the right side of the heart and enter the pulmonary circulation where they block arteries to the lungs and deprive areas of the lung of circulation (*pulmonary embolism*). If the obstruction involves a large pulmonary artery, large segments of lung may be involved *(pulmonary infarction)* causing chest pain, shortness of breath, cough, bloody sputum, and occasionally shock and death. Deep thrombophlebitis is more apt to cause this serious complication than is superficial thrombophlebitis.

Because of the danger of pulmonary embolism and infarction, thrombophlebitis is treated with bed rest and elevation of the affected extremity. Anticoagulants, or blood thinners, are given to decrease venous thrombus formation. In patients who have conditions that predispose them to the development of thrombophlebitis—such as a myocardial infarction, severe trauma requiring prolonged bed rest, or prolonged unconsciousness—anticoagulants are often prescribed to prevent the development of thrombophlebitis. In patients who have already experienced a pulmonary infarction or have had repeated bouts of thrombophlebitis, lifelong anticoagulation may be necessary.

The diagnosis of thrombophlebitis can be confirmed by ultrasound (Doppler technique) or by the injection of a radiopaque dye into the veins of the foot and taking serial radiographs. This technique, called *phlebography*, allows visualization of the veins of the legs to detect the presence of thrombi. The diagnosis of pulmonary infarction can be confirmed in some cases by chest radiography but may require a lung scan or an arteriogram of the pulmonary arteries for definite diagnosis. If history, physical examination, and initial tests raise suspicion of pulmonary embolism, a lung scan will usually confirm or dismiss that diagnosis.

*Varicose veins* are tortuous, dilated, superficial veins that usually occur in the lower extremities and are caused by impaired venous return. The underlying cause of varicose veins may be incompetence of the venous valves that normally prevent backflow of venous blood. Weaknesss of the wall of the vein may be another factor leading to varicose veins. Unlike deep thrombophlebitis, varicosities do not pose a threat of pulmonary emboli and infarction. They may give rise to a dull aching type of pain. Surgical removal is often done for cosmetic reasons.

# Diseases of the Aorta and Peripheral Vascular System

**Leriche's Syndrome (Aortoiliac Obstruction)** Atherosclerosis obstructs blood flow to the lower abdominal aorta just above its division into the two iliac arteries that supply the lower extremities with blood. The interference with the supply of blood and oxygen frequently results in pain in the hips and thighs, especially with exercise. If the obstruction is complete, gangrene may develop. Surgical repair by graft replacement is the treatment of choice.

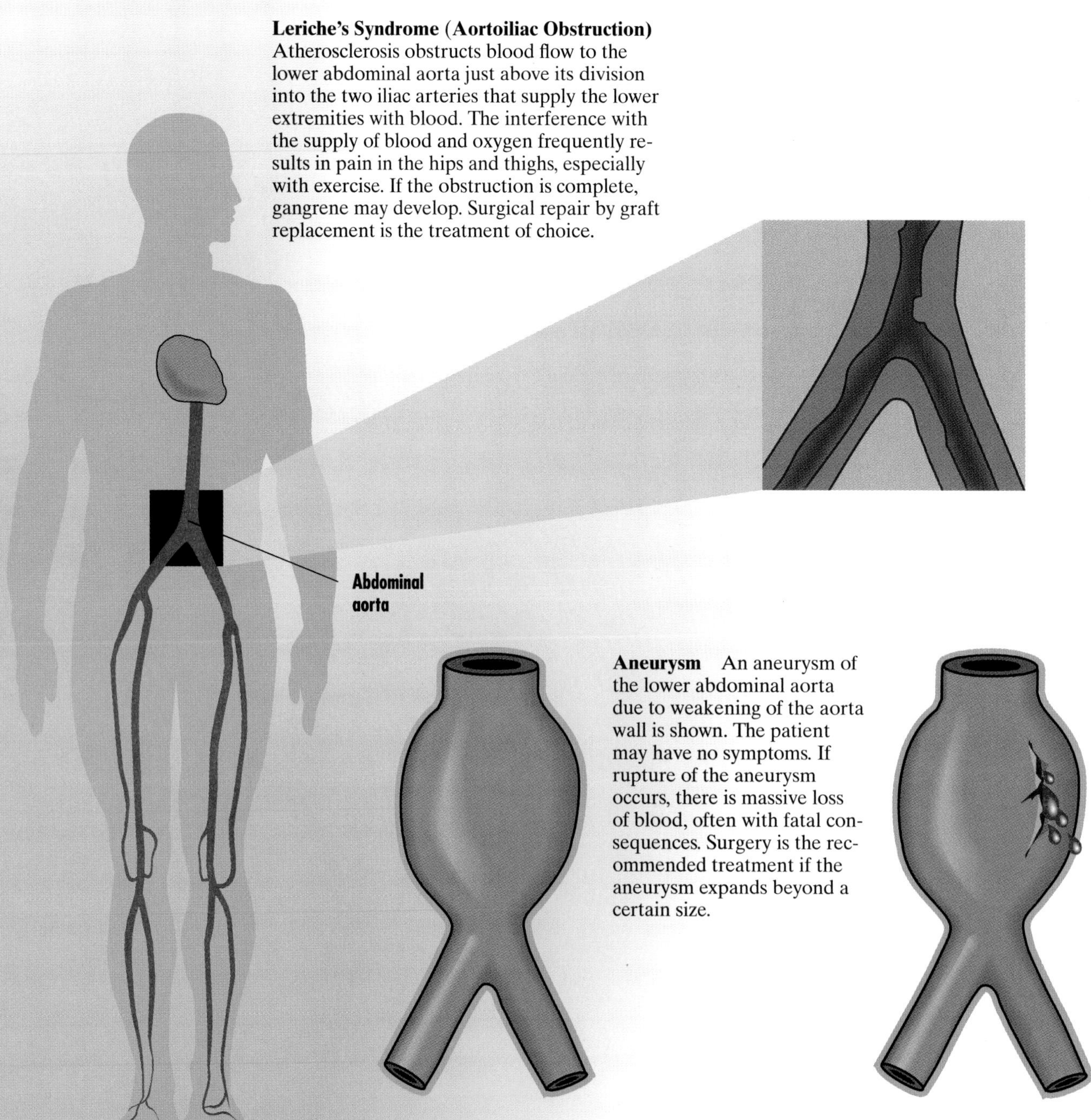


**Aneurysm** An aneurysm of the lower abdominal aorta due to weakening of the aorta wall is shown. The patient may have no symptoms. If rupture of the aneurysm occurs, there is massive loss of blood, often with fatal consequences. Surgery is the recommended treatment if the aneurysm expands beyond a certain size.

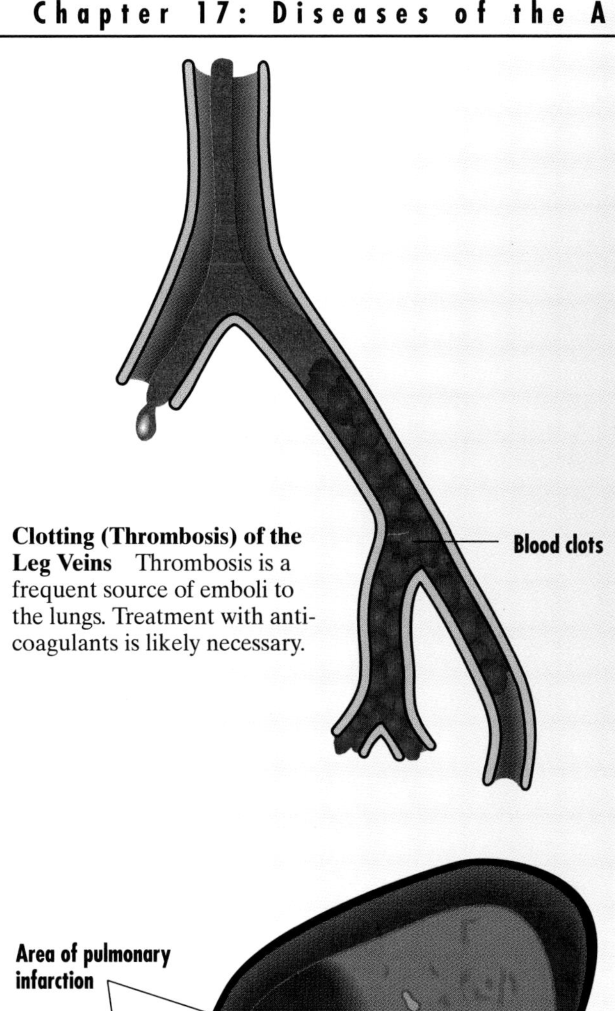


**Clotting (Thrombosis) of the Leg Veins** Thrombosis is a frequent source of emboli to the lungs. Treatment with anticoagulants is likely necessary.

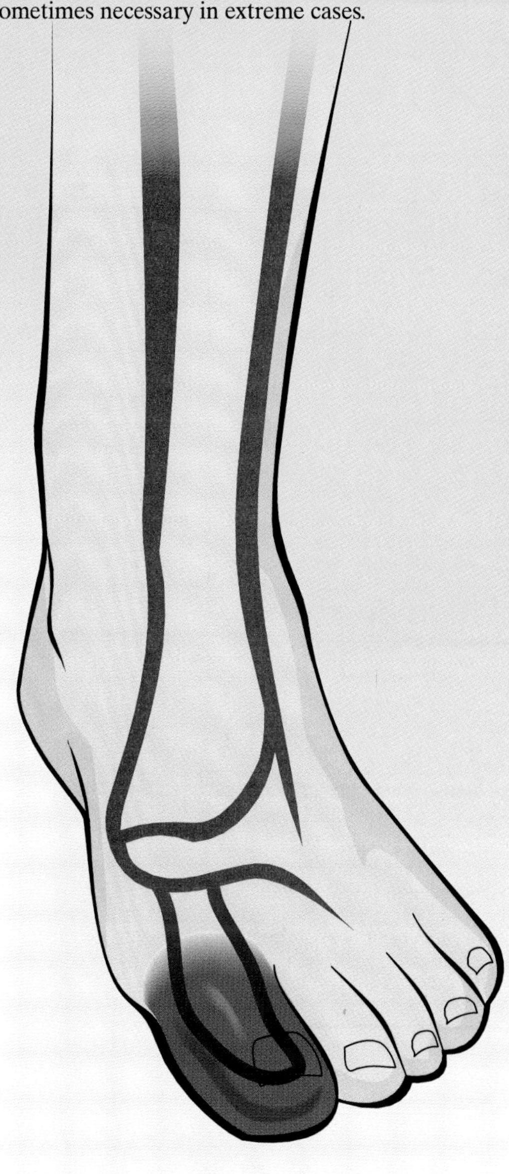

**Gangrene** An insufficient blood supply to the great toe, caused by a blocked artery, leads to gangrene. The blockage is usually associated with arteriosclerosis of the blood vessels of the affected leg. Amputation is sometimes necessary in extreme cases.

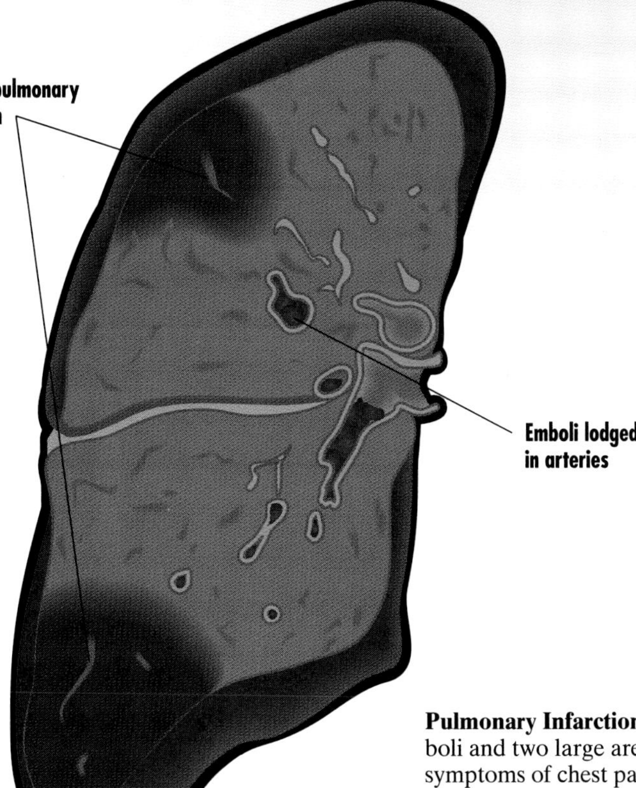


**Pulmonary Infarction** This lung has multiple emboli and two large areas of infarction. Immediate symptoms of chest pain, cough, shortness of breath, along with serious impairment of lung function may be the result of such a condition.

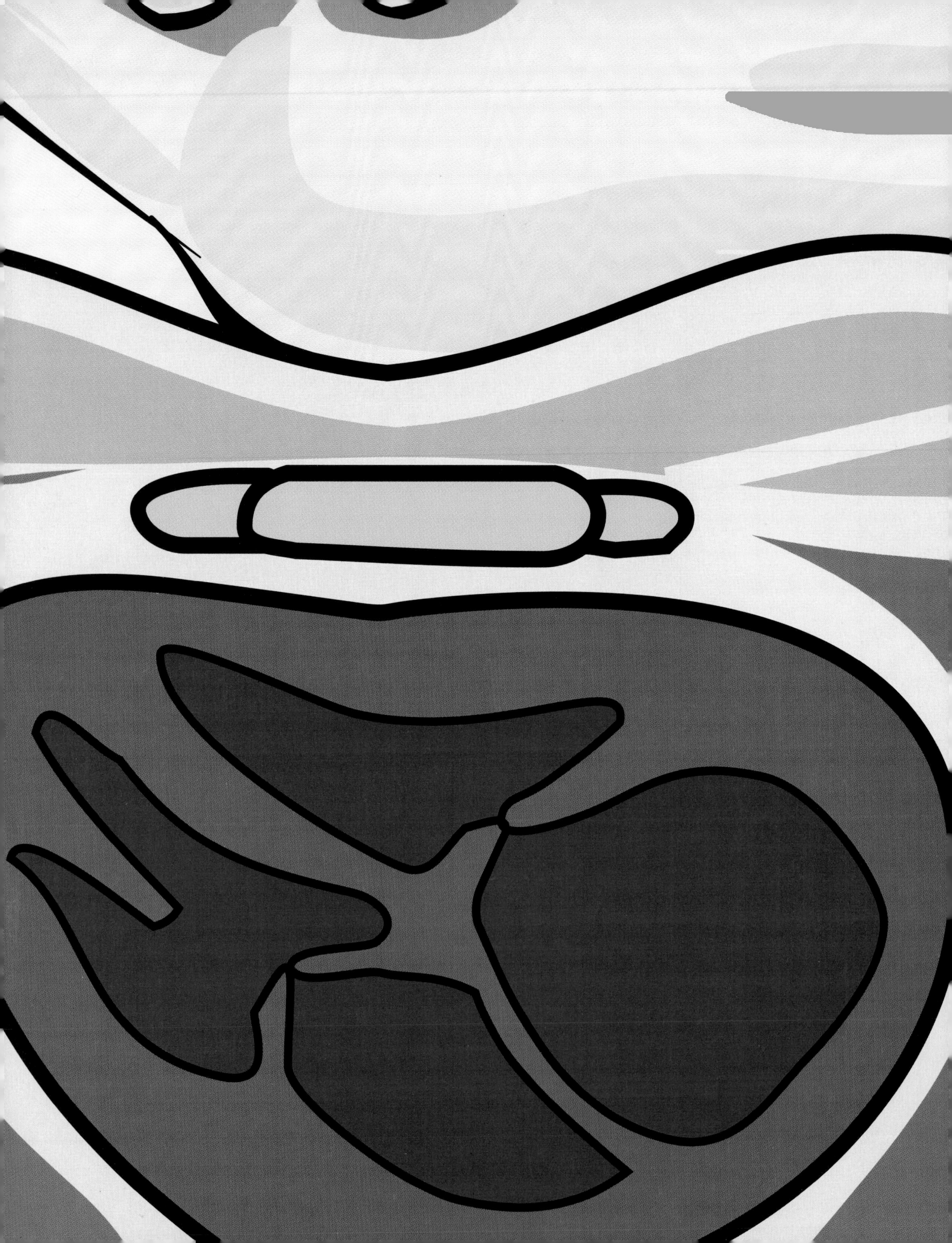

# 6 CARDIOPULMONARY RESUSCITATION (CPR)

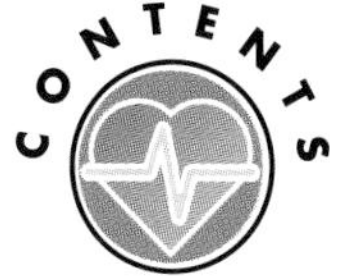

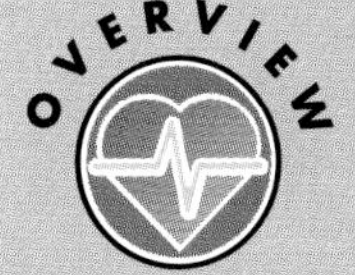
OVERVIEW

IN PARTS 1 THROUGH 5 of *How Your Heart Works,* we have discussed the normal and abnormal aspects of the heart and the vascular system. In Chapter 18 we will deviate from this pattern to present the topic of cardiopulmonary resuscitation (CPR), a basic life-support method. Despite its remarkable properties that we have previously reviewed, the heart is not indestructible. Under certain circumstances, it fails, and unless there is help from "the outside," the results are fatal.

Cardiopulmonary resuscitation is one of the most important of all emergency medical procedures. If a person's heart and lungs fail and cease to function—a situation called cardiopulmonary arrest—CPR is essential in avoiding the damage to the brain that begins 4 to 6 minutes after cessation of heart and lung action. The aim of CPR is to establish circulation and ventilation that will provide adequate oxygen to vital organs such as the brain and heart until those organs are able to function again on their own.

Immediate CPR may make the difference between life and death for victims of ischemic heart disease and acute myocardial infarction. It is also valuable for victims of drowning, electrocution, drug intoxication, suffocation, and serious accidents.

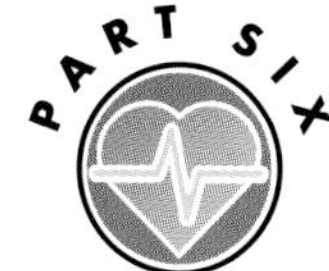


The time constraints that prevail in cardiopulmonary arrest do not allow for the arrival of professional rescue personnel. Each year in the United States there are about 640,000 deaths from ischemic heart disease. Of those, approximately 350,000 deaths occur outside hospitals, and most of these occur within a few minutes, in the presence of relatives, friends, and coworkers. It is plain to see that the training of nonmedical personnel in CPR is critical.

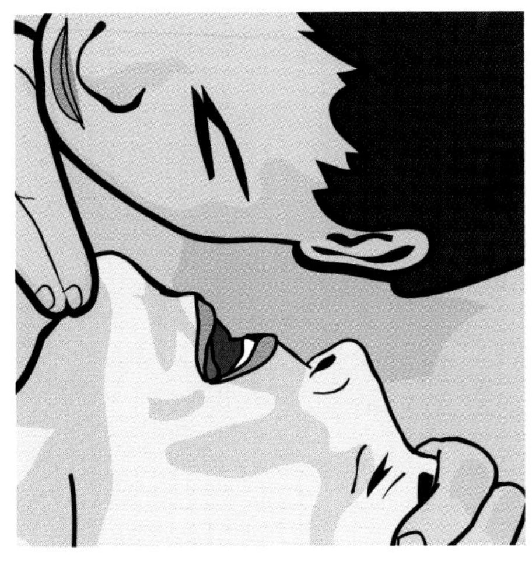

# When and How to Do CPR

THE NEED FOR immediate emergency life-support assistance—cardiopulmonary resuscitation or CPR—is usually obvious in victims of electrocution, drowning, suffocation, and serious accidents. Under other circumstances and until proved otherwise, an unconscious person should always be considered to have had cessation of heart and lung (pulmonary) function, referred to as *cardiopulmonary arrest.* Efforts should be made to obtain help from professionally trained medical assistance teams in the area, including the police. The management of such an emergency situation involves several steps.

First, make sure the person is actually unconscious: Some persons who appear to be unconscious actually may be sleeping or resting. If the person does not respond to stimulation such as shaking, shouting, or pain, he or she should be considered unconscious and a potential candidate for CPR.

Second, the victim must be lying on his or her back, and on a straight, firm surface for CPR to be administered effectively. If the victim has been in an accident and is likely to have sustained internal or neck injuries or fractures, extreme care must be exercised in getting the person into position.

Third, the rescuer must be aware of and adhere closely to the ABC of cardiopulmonary resuscitation principles—*airway, breathing,* and *circulation.*

**Airway** The airway of every unconscious person must be open so that there is free access of air to the victim's lungs. In an unconscious patient, the tongue usually falls back in the throat, causing airway obstruction. Accidentally inhaled objects such as pieces of toys or large pieces of food may also obstruct the airway. The head-tilt/chin-lift method is the safest maneuver to use to open the airway. The rescuer places one hand on the victim's forehead. The fingers of the rescuer's other hand are placed under the bony part of the lower jaw, near the chin. The rescuer then tilts the head back and lifts the jaw. Avoid closing the victim's mouth and pushing on the soft parts under the chin. Lifting the neck should also be avoided because of the danger of worsening a possible neck injury.

**Breathing** The victim should be checked for the presence of respiration. This can be done by observing the chest for signs of breathing motions or by placing one's ear close to the victim's mouth, then carefully listening and feeling for exhalation of air. In some cases, opening the airway is sufficient to initiate breathing. In the absence of spontaneous breathing, assisted mouth-to-mouth breathing should be initiated. The rescuer maintains the open airway of the victim, and with the thumb and forefinger of the hand on the victim's forehead, pinches closed the victim's nostrils so that air cannot escape through the nose. The rescuer than places his or her mouth over the victim's mouth, forming a tight seal. The rescuer takes a deep breath and exhales completely into the victim's mouth. This procedure is repeated 2 times to expand the victim's lungs, which are probably in a collapsed state. Thereafter, exhalations should be given at the rate of about 12 per minute. The rescuer must evaluate adequacy of the mouth-to-mouth respirations by sensing any resistance to the exhalations, and by observing movement of the victim's chest wall in response to the exhalations. If there is evidence of continuing airway obstruction, efforts should be repeated to clear it.

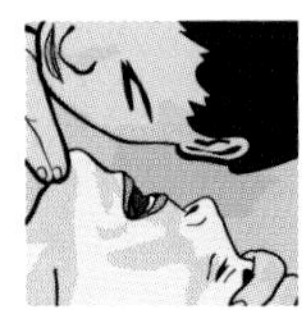

**Circulation** Palpation of the carotid arteries in the neck is the most convenient and reliable method of determining the presence of heart contractions. If there is no pulse present, external chest compression must be initiated. The rescuer kneels next to the victim's chest midway between the shoulder and the waist. The lower tip of the breastbone (sternum) is located with the index and middle fingers of one hand, the palpating hand. The other hand is placed on the sternum next to and just overlapping the index finger of the palpating hand. The palpating hand is now removed and the heel of this hand placed on top of the other hand. Chest compression is now begun. The object of each compression is to depress the sternum 1 to 1½ inches, thereby squeezing the heart between the sternum and the spine. Chest compressions should be done at the rate of about 1 per second, of which ½ second is used for compression and ½ second for relaxation. A convenient way to approximate this schedule is by repeating "one one thousand, two one thousand, three one thousand, four one thousand, five one thousand," and compressing the chest on "one, two, three, four, and five."

If the rescuer is alone, 15 compressions should be alternated with 2 ventilations. With the help of a second rescuer, one person can maintain compression and the other can maintain ventilation (5 compressions, then a ventilation). Switching positions to combat fatigue should be done without interruption of the CPR rhythm. Spontaneous breathing and return of pulse should be checked about every minute by the person performing mouth-to-mouth breathing.

Cardiopulmonary resuscitation should be continued until professional rescue help arrives or the victim initiates spontaneous heart and lung action.

# How to Perform CPR

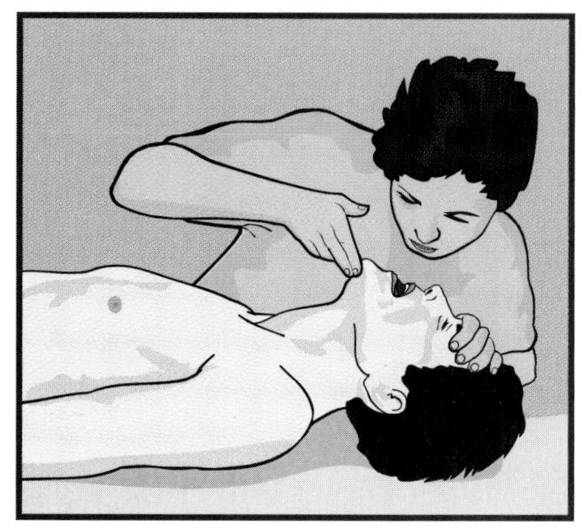

**Open the Airway** The head-tilt/chin-lift method is the safest maneuver to use to open the airway. The rescuer places one hand on the victim's forehead. The fingers of the rescuer's other hand are placed under the bony part of the lower jaw, near the chin. The rescuer then tilts the head and lifts the jaw. Avoid closing the victim's mouth and pushing on the soft parts under the chin. Lifting the neck should also be avoided because of the danger of worsening a possible neck injury.

**Check for Signs of Breathing** The rescuer listens and feels for evidence of breathing.

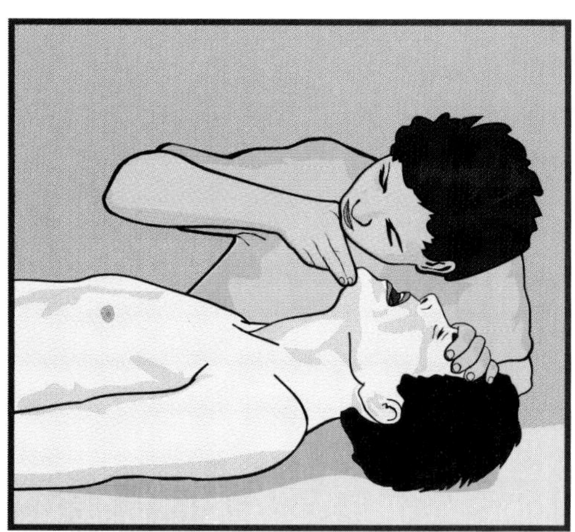

## The A, B, and C of Basic Life Support

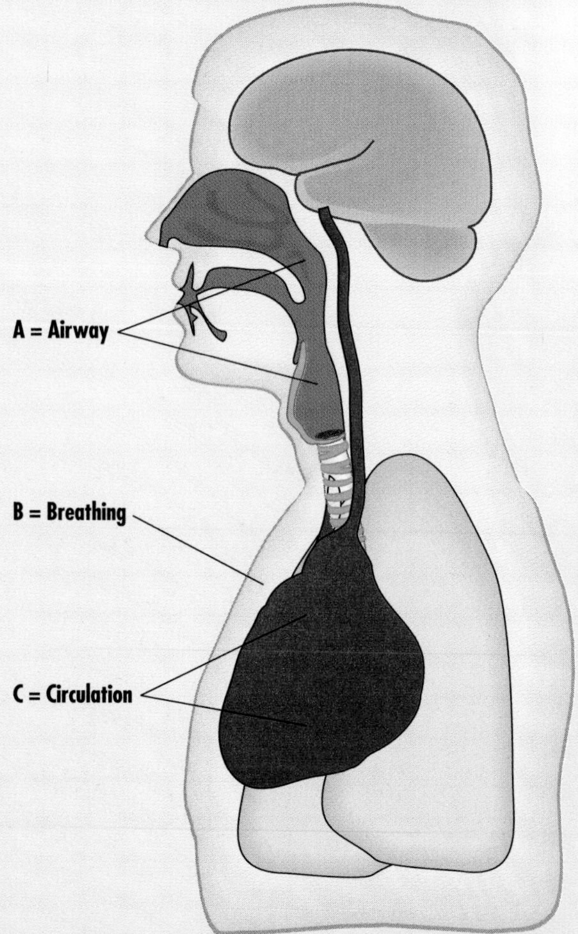


**Administer Mouth-to-Mouth Breathing** The rescuer maintains the open airway by pressing down on the victim's forehead with one hand, then pinches the victim's nose shut. The rescuer then forms a tight seal between his or her mouth and the mouth of the victim. Two full breaths are administered. Thereafter, exhalations should be administered at the rate of 12 per minute.

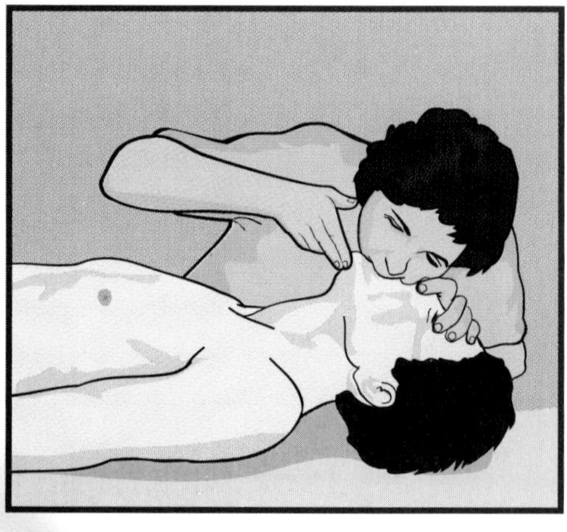

# Performing External Chest Compression

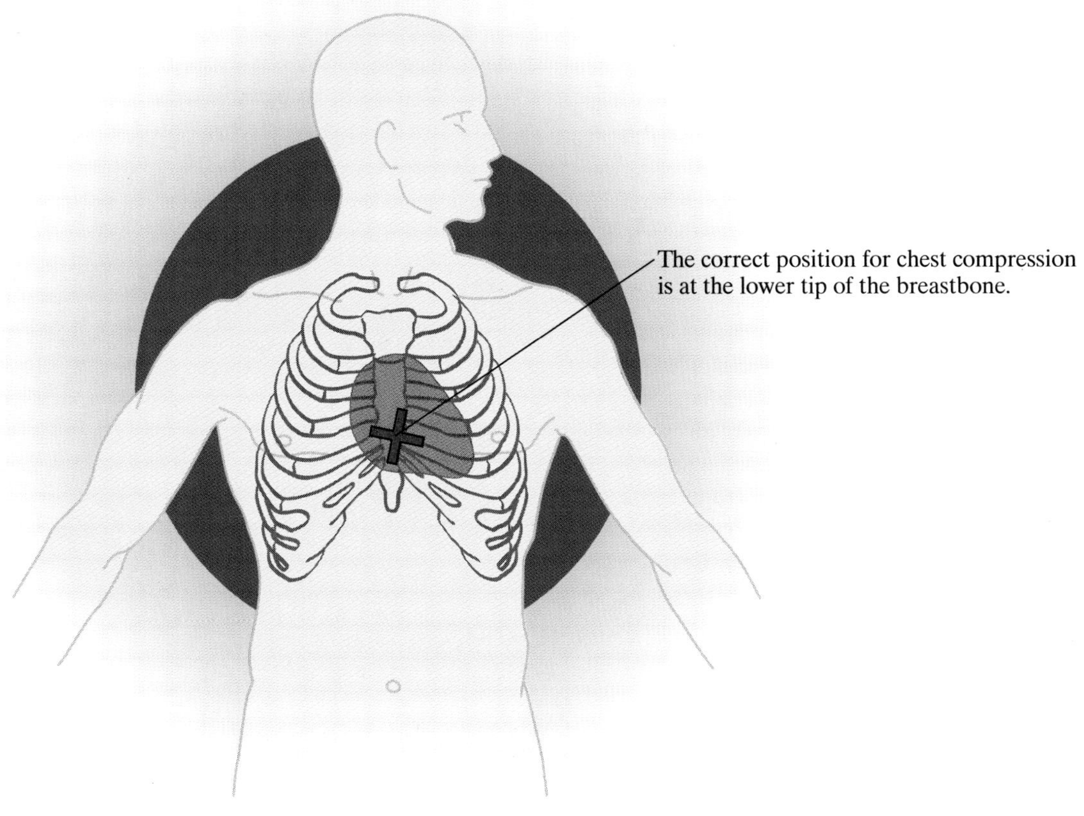


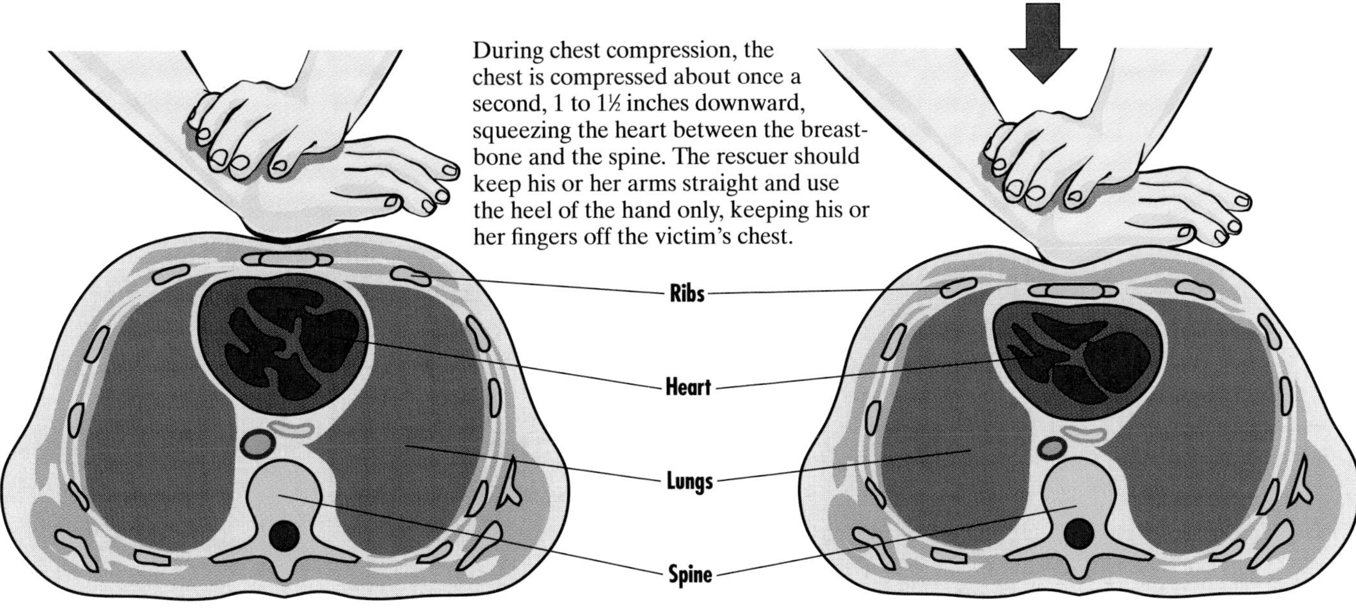

## P



## Q



## R